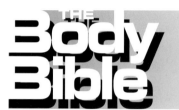

The Body Bible

BY PETA BEE

Written by Peta Bee
Design: Alan Hunns
Photographer: Dan Smith
Published by SportsBooks Limited
PO Box 422A
Surbiton
Surrey
KT5 9YP
United Kingdom

e-mail:
bodybible@sportsbooks.ltd.uk

Printed in the UK by Biddles Limited

ISBN
1 899807 05 5

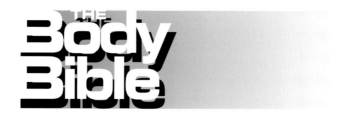

THE Body Bible

Peta Bee is the leading writer of the new fitness boom.

She contributes regularly to the award winning Style section of The Sunday Times as well as writing for The Express, Daily Mail, The Times, Daily Telegraph and Evening Standard. She also writes for Marie Claire, Health and Beauty, Health and Fitness, Top Sante and GQ Active magazines among others.

A graduate in Sports Science from Carnegie College, Leeds Metropolitan University, Peta is 31 and lives in London.

INTRODUCTION

Over the past 18 months, in the name of fitness, I have swallowed gallons of polluted water, played football with England coach Kevin Keegan and sailed in a yacht across the tarmac of a disused airport runway in Cambridgeshire. I have performed press-ups with my cat, a shimmy dance (of sorts) with the cast of a West End show and had a 12st man stand on my knees while I sat cross-legged on the floor. There have been occasions when I have returned home so battle-weary, that I have lacked the energy to plug in the kettle and been too full of aches and bruises to sit down. But I have had a ball.

That is not to say that I have enjoyed every single activity I have tried. Some I have finished and vowed never to do again, others I have thought to be pointless fun. Yet what I learned from doing all of them is that no one activity suits everyone, but search around and there will be one that suits you. The key is not to get disheartened if you try something that doesn't work for you. Persevere and you will stumble across an activity that will leave you feeling as if you have just stepped off the Olympic rostrum. This book is intended merely as a guide to point you in the right direction. Only through trying a range of activities yourself will you discover which one lights your flame.

For me it was something as simple as riding a bike. Yes, I could do it by the time I was six, alright, and at great speed as I recall. But at the age of 11 I was routinely entered for my Cycling Proficiency test, an obligatory afternoon of scrutiny in West Midlands primary schools in the late 1970s, and my early love affair with the bicycle came to an emergency stop. I became the only pupil in the history of my school to be deemed unroadworthy by the examiners. This apparent injustice punctured my ego and it remained a skeleton in my closet that has routinely been bought out to haunt me, much to the hilarity of friends and family, over the years. While my class mates were each awarded a signed certificate in the school assembly, all I got was a hand-written note from my headmaster, Mr Middleton, encouraging me to "keep on cycling."

Needless to say, I didn't. It took almost two decades and one almighty leap of faith to get me back on two wheels again. It was only when I agreed to take part in an adventure race which required me to complete part of the course on bicycle that I made my comeback. It was a shaky return and I lagged somewhat behind my team-mates, but as achievements go that one left me feeling pretty chuffed. I have since invested in a mountain bike and go off-road riding on a regular basis and, although I doubt whether I would pass my cycling proficiency test even today, I can state, hand on heart, that I enjoy free-wheeling along the cycle paths of Richmond Park. Which is more than I, and presumably Mr Middleton, could ever have hoped for.

And that in a nutshell is the underlying theme of The Body Bible. For any form of physical activity to be worthwhile, it must be something that rewards you with a sense of achievement and a feeling of well-being. Likewise, your reasons for doing it in the first place should be positive. Try any of the sports or exercise classes in these pages if they take your fancy, if you want to prove to yourself that you can or if you think they will inspire you to try bigger and better things. Dip in and out of each chapter. But above all have fun as you get fitter.

And finally, don't let lingering doubts about your capabilities or irrational fears about a particular activity get in your way. We all have dreams, but more often than not it is our reluctance to act on them that proves the biggest stumbling block in preventing us achieving what we want. You might have thought about running a marathon, taking up karate, learning to swim or in-line skating through the stationary traffic to work each morning. So what's stopping you? Whatever your personal fitness goal, if you want it badly enough, it's yours.

Why Keep Fit?

Scientists have proven that a life of inertia is not the route to health and happiness. Regular exercise, they say, improves body image and self-esteem, reduces stress and helps ward off a range of killer diseases.

In research it has been shown that exercising for longer than 20 minutes at a time triggers the production of endorphins, the body's natural feel-good chemicals, from the brain, leaving you on an emotional high. And then there are the proven medical benefits. Regular physical activity will help you to replace excess body fat with toned muscle as you lose weight. This reduces the risk of you becoming obese which is a risk factor for many conditions like diabetes, heart disease and strokes. Over time, exercise will strengthen the cardiovascular system, enabling your heart and lungs to work more efficiently, and will also improve circulation. According to the British Heart Foundation around 10,000 deaths from heart attacks could be prevented each year if people kept themselves fitter.

Weekly periods of inertia are thought to be one reason why obesity levels are rising in the UK. The Health Survey for England carried out in 1999 revealed that 20 per cent of women and 17 per cent of men are now obese compared with only eight per cent of women and six per cent of men in 1980. Similarly, Department of Health figures show that there has been four per cent rise in the number of women who are clinically obese since 1995, all of which further increases the risks of high blood pressure, heart disease and strokes.

Exercise is also important in the prevention of osteoporosis, the bone-thinning disease which affects one in three women and one in 12 men at some time in their lives. The National Osteoporosis Society recently launched a campaign to raise awareness of the benefits that weight-bearing exercise, such as walking, jogging and aerobics, can have on building bone strength. Exercise will also boost flexibility, balance, spatial awareness and reaction times all of which have a positive knock-on effect in other areas of life such as work.

Yet, despite the proven benefits, most of us still don't break into a sweat or raise ourselves off the couch often enough. A 1997 Hansbro report showed that one quarter of all adults (that is 24 per cent of men and 26 per cent of women) aged 16 to 74 are sedentary, meaning they do less than half an hour of moderate intensity physical activity each week. A staggering six out of ten men and seven out of ten women don't do enough exercise to benefit their health.

A 1999 study showed that we are particularly sedentary at weekends. Researchers at Loughborough University interviewed over 150 adults about their regular exercise levels. After six months of the year-long study, it was found that subjects slipped into inactivity mode every Friday. Sustained regular activity is considered far more effective at keeping off the pounds than a regular burn-out at the gym.

The Health Education Authority's (HEA) guidelines suggest that half an hour of moderate exercise every day is enough to keep in shape. Previously it was thought that three 20 minute sessions of vigorous activity per week were required to maintain minimum fitness, but it is now known that a cumulative amount of lower intensity exercise is just as good for your health. The HEA recommends walking as one of the best forms of physical exercise, claiming that newcomers to exercise who begin walking for half an hour every day will soon halve their risk of heart disease.

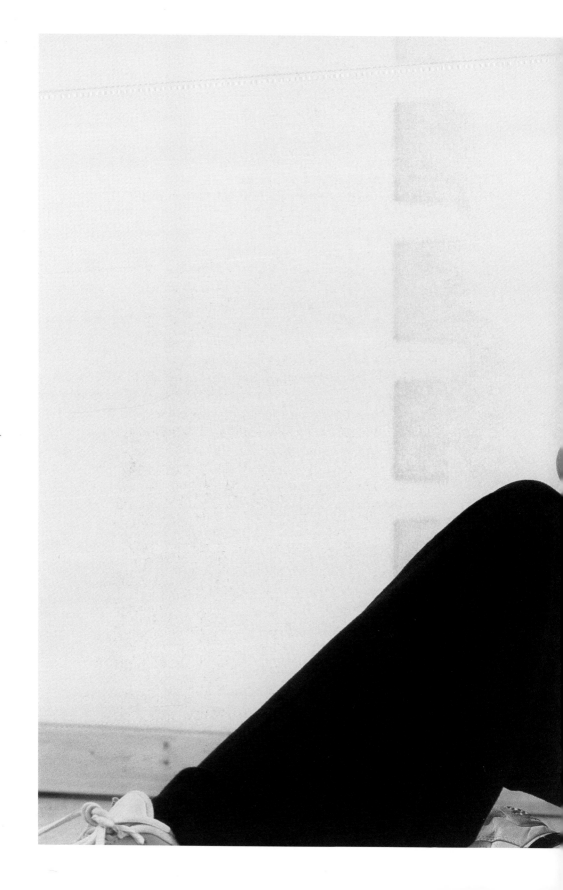

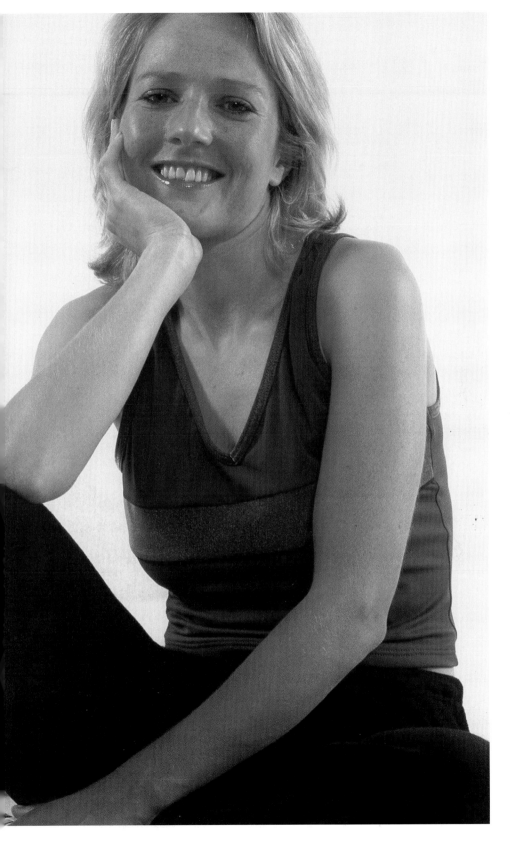

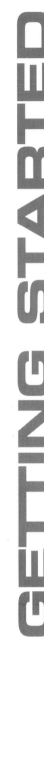
GETTING STARTED

Peta: "I've had a ball."

GETTING STARTED

How fit are you?

Assessing your fitness level on a regular basis is one of the best ways to motivate yourself into keeping up the good work. If you can see progress, you are more likely to carry on; if you can see decline, you may be inspired to exercise a little more frequently or at a higher intensity.

Real fitness is not a matter of measuring how long you can keep going on the treadmill, it is a combination of all-round physiological benefits that leave you fit enough to live life to the full. According to sports physiologists, there are numerous ways to assess how fit you are as part of your on-going workout regime. The tests below will give an idea of where you are at in specific aspects of fitness and will help you to pinpoint which areas need extra attention. Warm up thoroughly before attempting the tests and perform them once every six weeks if you can. Keep a record of your progress so that you can see how you are improving.

The step test

This tests for cardiovascular fitness. You will need a bench, sturdy box or step about eight to ten inches high. Check your heart rate before you start by taking your pulse for 15 seconds and multiplying the figure by four to give you a one minute figure. Keeping your back straight, hands on hips and abdominal muscles tucked in, begin stepping up and down from the box. Keep upright – don't lean forward. Maintain a steady but fast pace for two minutes, aiming to take about 40 steps per minute. Sit down and take your pulse again. Subtract the first figure from the second figure – what is the difference?

(a) Less than ten beats a minute – indicates a good level of aerobic fitness.
(b) Ten beats a minute – average aerobic fitness.
(c) More than ten beats a minutes – below average aerobic fitness.

The strength test

Strong muscles not only look good, but they are important for supporting the skeleton and maintaining good posture. How many consecutive push-ups/press-ups can you manage to perform without taking a rest?

(a) Less than five – low strength levels.
(b) Five to ten – average strength.
(c) More than ten – good strength.

Speed test

Make sure you warm up thoroughly before this test. On flat ground measure out 20 metres in a straight line (about 20 medium length paces). Ask someone to time you while you run the distance at top speed. What is your time?

(a) Eight seconds or more – too slow.
(b) Five to eight seconds – reasonable pace.
(c) Less than five seconds – fast pace.

Flexibility test

For any fitness programme and for daily life in general, it is important that you maintain a good level of flexibility so that you can move muscles through a full range around joints. Try this test to see how flexible you are in your hamstring muscles and lower back: Sit on the floor with legs together and directly out in front of you. Your bottom and back should be against a wall or door. Slowly lean forward towards your toes. How far can you reach with your fingertips?

(a) To your knees – poor flexibility.
(b) Between your knees and ankles – reasonable flexibility.
(c) To your ankles or beyond – excellent flexibility.

Muscular Endurance

Test how long your muscles can keep working at an intense level with this simple test. Stand with your back against a wall and move your body down and feet out until your knees are bent at right angles to the floor. Maintain that position for as long as you can. How long can you sit there?

(a) Less than 30 seconds – poor strength endurance.
(b) Between 30 seconds and one minute – reasonable strength endurance.
(c) More than one minute – excellent strength endurance.

Body Mass Index (BMI)

Your BMI is a widely used means of assessing whether or not you are overweight. It is not a definitive test but is considered more accurate than the old height and weight charts. Divide your weight in kilograms by your height in metres squared. For example, if you weigh 60 kg and are 1.7 metres tall, your BMI will be 60 divided by 2.9 = 20.5 (round up or down to the nearest 0.5).

What is yours?

(a) Thirty plus – too heavy.
(b) Between 25 and 30 – average to slightly overweight.
(c) Between 20 and 25 – ideal weight.

New health index:

Divide your waist measurement by your height; above 0.5 increased risk; above 0.6 substantially increased risk. Eg: waist measurement of 82 cm (0.82metres) divided by height measurement of 1.95 metres is 0.42.

BUYING KIT

Walk into any high street sports shop and the dazzling array of equipment on offer can fool you into thinking you need to spend a small fortune to get kitted out for sport. In fact, the basics can be bought relatively inexpensively. Comfort and breathability should be the main things you look for in exercise gear, so make sure you try on everything before you buy. If possible, stretch or at least walk around to check that it allows full range of movement and doesn't rub or ride up and down. Always look for garments with covered seams and padded straps to avoid chaffing.

If you are planning to exercise indoors, then look for stretchy fabrics that contain a percentage of the elastic fabric, Lycra. Tights, thigh-length shorts, leotards, crop tops and vests are available in a range of mix-and-match colour-ways. For swimming, opt for lightweight Lycra swimsuits rather than fashion garments which tend to be made from heavier fabrics and can increase drag which will slow you down. A good-quality, well-fitting pair of goggles is a must as is a hat if you have long hair. Always rinse swimsuits out in cold water as soon as you leave the pool because chlorine rots the Lycra fabric.

The golden rule for any outdoor activity is to layer, layer, layer. Several lightweight base layers will not only keep you warmer than a heavyweight sweatshirt or fleece as air will be trapped between the garments, but it is also easier to peel off one piece of clothing at a time and wrap it round your waist as you warm up. Most of the big sportswear manufacturers now produce sweat-wicking fabrics that are designed to keep moisture away from the skin as you work out – Nike has DRI-FIT, adidas has Climalite etc. These are comfortable and wash well, so are worth the initially higher financial outlay compared with conventional fabrics. Cotton, for example, tends to soak up and store sweat causing the skin to become clammy and cold if it is worn for any length of time during vigorous exercise.

For some sports it is best to visit a specialist shop where you will get specific advice about equipment to suit your needs. For running or jogging you will need a loose-fitting pair of shorts, a vest or t-shirt and some lightweight, seam-free socks to lessen the risk of blistering. Cyclists will need to invest in a good quality helmet that meets safety standards, a water bottle, a puncture kit and some padded cycling shorts. A small hip-bag that fastens around the waist is useful for keeping small change and other essentials when you are venturing a few miles from home.

As with any wardrobe, it is best to buy the basic sports wear and add more garments if and when you decide you need them. For women a good sports bra is essential (see page 19). Otherwise both men and women should invest in a warm, loose fitting tracksuit with pockets, some good quality training shoes (see below) and a showerproof or waterproof jacket for starters. Breathable waterproof fabrics, like GoreTex, allow sweat to evaporate through tiny pores in the fabric but also have a special waterproof coating that ensures the clothing next to your skin stays dry. They are expensive but hard-wearing and if you care for them properly will last for years.

TRAINERS

Inconceivable as it seems, 20 years ago it was only the seriously sporty who would have considered buying a pair of trainers. Now, however, they are uniquely marketed as being both high-fashion and high-comfort enough for the young, old, lumpy and bumpy to wear. Fuelled by manufacturers' advertising campaigns which tell us how their latest high-tech, all-singing, all-dancing trainer is the best favour we can do for our feet, we continue to buy them in our droves. The UK market for the humble running shoe now exceeds £175million with more than four million pairs sold every year.

Yet experts are not so sure that this is money wisely spent. According to podiatrists and chiropodists who treat people with foot injuries, sometimes trainers are actually harmful for our feet. Ill-fitting and worn-out sports shoes that have seen better days can cause anything from a niggle to acute pain and even long term damage. Simon Costain, a podiatrist at the Harley Street Gait and Posture Clinic, says the most common are caused by wearing trainers with too little support on the upper which results in feet pronating, or rolling inwards, further than they should. This can result in lower back ache, hip pain, runner's knee, shin pain and problems on the arch and ball of the foot.

A sports shoe can even have too much cushioning. When you run or jump, each time your foot strikes the ground it absorbs the force of four times your own body weight which reverberates up through the legs and into the spine. There is little doubt that a spongy shoe helps to absorb much of the shock and prevent related injuries. But shoes with a high degree of cushioning are only necessary for people with high arches on their feet, about five per cent of the population says Simon Costain. For the rest of us, too much sponginess means too much unnecessary movement. Your feet can literally wobble out of control.

And as attached as you feel to the trusty old Nike Air or adidas trainers you have been jogging in since the year dot, there comes a time when you must put emotions aside and accept that they are probably doing you more harm than good. "Trainers have a shelf-life of six months to one year, depending on how often you use them, but you should definitely replace them after running a total of 500 miles," says podiatric surgeon Trevor Prior. "If you've had a pair for longer than that, the best place for them is the bin." If you are prone to foot pain of any sort, it is worth consulting a registered podiatrist who will be able to advise you on the most suitable design of shoe for your feet.

How much should you spend?

Investing a small fortune in your trainers won't necessarily ensure you get a better constructed shoe. A 1997 study published in the British Journal of Sports Medicine investigated the deceptive advertising claims of running shoes. Researchers rigorously assessed the merits of a wide range of trainers and concluded that the more you pay for sports shoes, the more likely you are to get injured. "There are a lot of gimmicks at the more expensive end of the sports shoe market and manufacturers make unjustified claims about them in many cases," says Simon Costain. "My advice would be not to opt for the cheapest shoe around but to choose a pair in the mid-price range of £60-£80. For your the sake of your feet, it is better value to buy two pairs of trainers at £60 than one high fashion pair at £120."

Are your trainers safe?

There are plenty of well-made trainers on the market and often it is consumer ignorance that has a part to play in trainer injuries. A common mistake is to buy trainers that are too small which constrict the toes and increase the risk of bruising on the toenails and heels. In general you will need a half size bigger in sports shoes than in regular footwear. Always try on new trainers in the afternoon when feet have swollen and, since feet swell further when you exercise, wear a reasonably thick pair of socks to find the best fit. Ideally your heel should fit snugly in the cup and the fit should be just tight enough not to allow any movement up and down or from side to side when you walk. Here, podiatrist Trevor Prior suggests a check list to tell if your trainers have passed their sell-by date:

Check that there is some tread left on the bottom of the shoe. If the pattern has worn away completely, it is time to invest in a new pair as protection will be reduced. Also look for more wear and tear on one side of the sole than the other which could affect your posture. The mid-sole cushioning, usually the white, spongier section of the shoe, should not be creased and flattened. If it is it provides limited cushioning for the feet and legs. This is often the area of a shoe which wears out first, so make sure you check regularly. If the fabric upper appears to slant in one direction, either inwards or outwards, it is a sign that your foot is also leaning inwards or outwards, leaving you prone to injury. Most reasonable quality trainers will have removable insoles. Check them regularly by removing them to see if they are worn away at the ball of the foot or the heel. This is a sign that your trainers have had their day.

Who to Contact: For a state registered podiatrist in your area, contact the Society of Chiropodists and Podiatrists (0207 486 3381) or consult the website at www.feetforlife.org; Simon Costain is at the Harley Street Gait and Posture Centre on 0207 636 4465; for an appointment with Trevor Prior call 0208 989 8252.

CHOOSING A SPORTS BRA

Fed up with jiggling uncontrollably beneath their t-shirts, back in 1977 two American women struck on the idea of sewing together a couple of jockstraps to provide support for their bouncing bosoms when they ran. Hence, the sports bra was conceived and the market for minimising bounce was born. Now sports science researchers are convinced that a well-constructed sports bra is essential for active women if they are to avoid their bosoms plummeting towards their feet.

A sports bra differs from an ordinary bra in a number of ways. It should be less elastic to restrict vertical movement and comes a little higher under the arms and at the front to hold the breasts well in against the chest wall. In research carried out for Berlei at Herriot Watt University, as many as 77 per cent of women who work out regularly don't wear a proper sports bra and almost one fifth wear no bra at all. Not only is this abandonment of performance underwear likely to increase feelings of discomfort during exercise, it can also cause lasting damage. In a study by the US Department of Exercise and Health, 20 women of varying bust dimensions were video-taped while jogging on a treadmill at a speed of 12km per hour. First they ran wearing no bra which caused their breasts to move an average 8.5cm up and down from their resting position. With the support of a ordinary bra, the women's breasts reduced the wobbling about by 32 per cent, but when they ran in a specialist sports bra, overall motion was restricted by a further 21 per cent.

Since breasts are made up of fat, not muscle, natural support is provided only by the skin that surrounds them and by the Cooper's ligaments that run from the nipples down to the pectoral muscles in the chest. Repetitive and high impact physical activity, like running, with an inadequate bra means the breasts bounce, stretching the fragile support system to its limits.

Over time the ligaments will lose their natural elasticity causing the breasts to sag irreversibly, something that can result in chronic back ache for heavier busted women.

So, for women who exercise, a well-fitting sports bra is as important an accessory as a well-fitting pair of shoes.

What's your size?

Research shows that around 85 per cent of all women in the UK wear the wrong sized bra – and that figure is thought to be much the same for women who exercise regularly. Ideally, you should go for a fitting and measurement at a specialist underwear outlet or even at a department store like Marks and Spencer. However, here is a guide to making sure you don't miscalculate your own vital statistics:

Chest dimension: Wearing an everyday bra, measure your rib cage directly beneath your breasts with a tape measure. Add five inches to the figure to find your chest dimension. If the total figure is an odd number like 33, then round it up to the next even number (34)

Bra Cup size: Hold the tape measure gently around the fullest part of your bust. Be careful not to pull too tightly as it will affect the result. If the measurement is one inch more than your chest dimension figure, then you are an A cup; 2 inches more means you are a B cup, three inches a C cup and so on.

Buying a sports bra

With the sports underwear market set to bust out all over this year, selecting the most suitable bra from the dizzying array on offer may be tricky. However, once you have sifted out the bra-tops designed to be worn over the top of sports bras and which offer insufficient support for your breasts during exercise, there are basically two types to choose from. Compression style bras, like the Minimal Bounce bra by Dans-Ez, work by holding the breast tissue in so that it gives an almost flattened appearance, while encapsulation sports bras, such as Berlei's Shock Absorbers, look more like a regular bra and work by surrounding (and cupping) the breast for support.

Here's a general guide to help you decide which you need
Small-breasted (cup sizes 32A/B to 34A) A compression bra will offer adequate support. Look for one made from sweat-wicking fabric with plenty of room beneath the arms to avoid chaffing when you run. Racer-style backs are a good choice if you have narrow shoulders as there is less likelihood of the straps slipping down.

Medium-breasted (cup sizes 34B to 36B) Although you might get away with wearing a compression-style bra for low impact types of exercise like weight training, you will need one of the more supportive encapsulation bras for running. Ideally choose one with individual cup sizes rather than simply opting for a small, medium or large sizing.

Large-breasted (cup size 36 C and bigger) An encapsulation bra is needed to support larger breasts in all forms of physical activity. Look for a wide band beneath the breast which will prevent the bra from rising upwards when you move. Cups should be well-fitting and support the entire breast. Straps should be fairly wide but preferably without too many seams or fastenings which can dig into or rub against the skin as you run.

JOINING A GYM

Joining a gym can be an expensive but worthwhile investment. Many gyms and health clubs offer top quality equipment, instruction and a range of classes held in safe, pleasant and sociable surroundings.

However, the standard of gyms and health clubs can vary enormously and it is worth visiting a few before making your choice.

Safety should be the number one consideration. In a 1997 Which? report, the Consumer's Association found that gyms were failing to give newcomers proper inductions, that seven out of ten aerobics sessions were badly taught and that some classes were even considered to be unsafe.

Even the rooms in which aerobics classes are held can pose a health risk. It is important, for instance, that a fitness class that involves a lot of bouncing and pounding is held in a room with sprung floors. Check, too, that fitness instructors are well-qualified – most should possess either an RSA, YMCA or NVQ certificate. If they don't it may be worthwhile looking elsewhere.

Check, too, that the gym meets your needs in terms of facilities. If you like swimming, make sure it has an adequately sized and well-maintained pool that is at least 25 metres long. Where the gym is situated is also important. For you to get your money's worth from the membership, the gym should be within easy access to your home or office.

How to check a gym is safe

Ask whether the gym you want to join offers a personal assessment of your diet, lifestyle, medical history and injuries. Ask whether the gym is affiliated to the Fitness Industry Association which requires its members to adhere to strict standards. Instructors should always explain how to use equipment and watch while you try out the apparatus. Make sure you are shown a thorough warm-up, stretch and cool down routine.

Check that rooms used for aerobics and other classes are well-ventilated or air-conditioned. Ask whether the room or studio has a sprung floor which will protect your joints against pounding. Some clubs display profiles of the instructors listing their qualifications. If this information isn't available, ask at the reception about the instructor's experience. Ask whether a gym limits its class sizes. An overcrowded class means less personal attention if you are having difficulties.

Who to Contact: Exercise England can advise you about where to go to contact a personal trainer or which qualifications to look for. Send an SAE to Exercise England, Solecast House, 13-27 Brunswick Place, London N1 6DX (0807 506506).

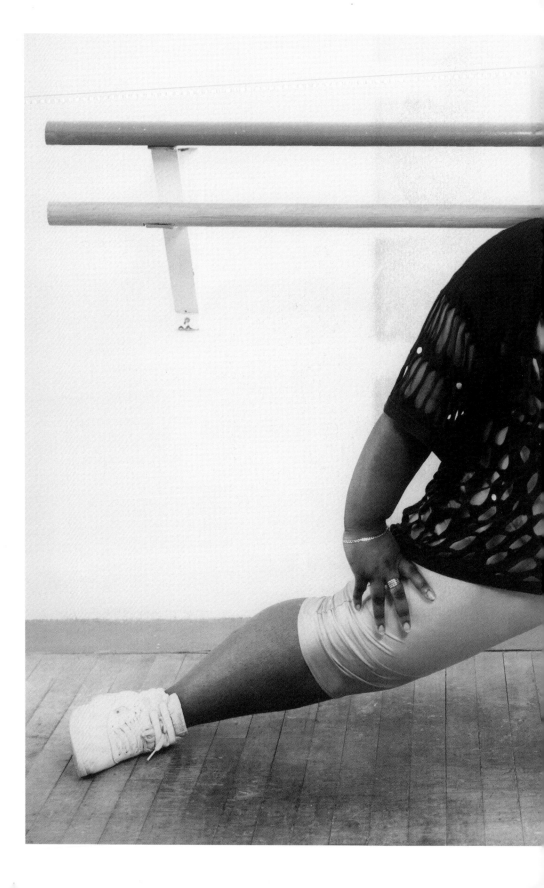

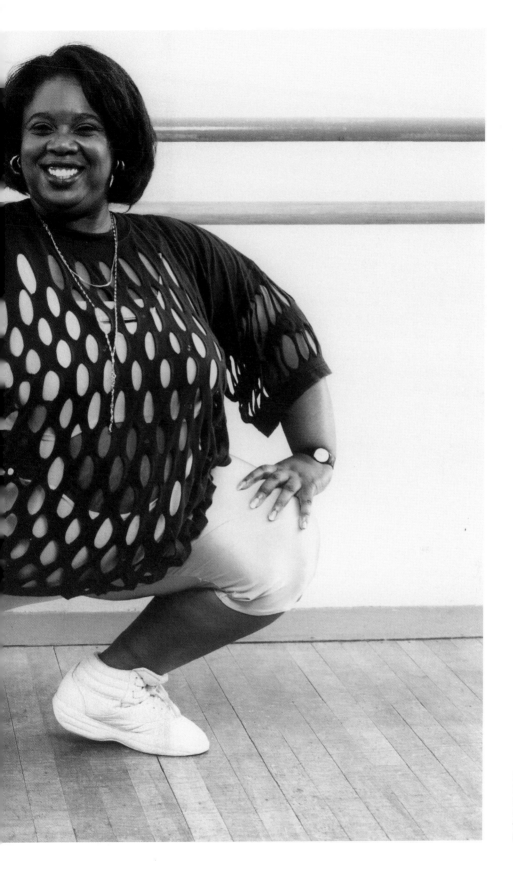

Instructor,
Kathryn
Szrodecki of
Great Shape
for Larger
Ladies

AEROBIC ACTIVITY

Aerobic exercise should always be the mainstay of any fitness programme. Basically, it is any form of activity which requires the body to increase its use of oxygen and while running, swimming and cycling are among the most popular aerobic activities, it encompasses everything from skipping to rowing and fitness classes.

When you work out aerobically your muscles require more oxygen than they would if you were standing still. The heart responds by pumping more blood which carries oxygen around the body. At first this is hard work, but the more aerobic training you do the more efficient your body becomes at using the oxygen supplies available. In time, the cardiovascular system also improves so that the heart can accomplish more work in the same amount of time.

After months of aerobic training your resting heart rate, your average number of heart beats per minute, will drop. This is a sign that your heart is pumping blood around the body more powerfully and efficiently than before.

But improved circulatory and cardiovascular systems are just one advantage of regular aerobic exercise. In conjunction with a healthy diet, is also considered the best and most effective way to reduce body fat and will boost your metabolism so that your body burns calories from food at a faster rate. And it is not just from running that you can hit the 'runner's high.'

Sports physiologists have shown that any form of aerobic exercise carried out for around 20 minutes triggers the release of feel-good chemicals that leave you feeling in a better mood than when you started.

The real beauty of aerobic exercise is that it can be done anywhere, inside or out. Ever since Jane Fonda bounded into our living rooms wearing leotard and leg-warmers in the early eighties, for gym-goers aerobic exercise has become synonymous with choreographed aerobic classes. While aerobics has its critics, its mass popularity is unwavering and over the last two decades the variety of classes has increased at least one hundred-fold and now there is literally one to suit every level of fitness.

The kind of high impact aerobics classes, first popularised by Fonda and those of the body burn school of thought, which involve a lot of pounding around have since become maligned with the tag of being dangerous for your knees.

But this is not necessarily the case. Like any new class, the key is not to dive into an advanced form of aerobics straight away because it will overload your joints and may cause problems.

Start off in low-impact classes, wear well-cushioned aerobics shoes which allow lateral and forward movement, not trainers, and don't push yourself out of your comfort zone are the golden rules in the early days. It also pays to check that your instructor is well-qualified, that the classes aren't over-crowded and that you are given a full warm-up and cool-down routine in every session.

In fact, it is more often the rooms where aerobics classes are held and not the exercise itself that predisposes people to injury. Make it a priority to check with your gym that it has sprung wooden floors in aerobics studios and that you won't be pounding up and down on rock solid surfaces.

In recent years, there have been numerous cases of employers being taken to court by aerobics instructors who have suffered injury to their knees and other joints after repeatedly teaching on hard, unsuitable floors.

BOOTCAMP WORKOUT

New Recruits to the Bootcamp class are taken aback when instructor Paul Sansome asks them to slip into combat gear on their arrival. And they look shell-shocked when he orders them to camouflage their faces with war paint before entering the dance studio at the left, quick march. If your body finds keeping fit enough of a battle at the best of times then the Bootcamp workout is not for you. By Sansome's reckoning, this military inspired workout is the equivalent of two aerobics sessions rolled into one torturous hour.

Adopting the role of sergeant major, Sansome makes it clear that he won't tolerate the weak-willed and can spot the sloucher who misses a press up even when his back is turned.

The class is based on a successful format from the US where it is a resounding success. Rather than just being another novelty workout, the entire routine is based on an exercise programme from the US army, which, says Sansome, makes it the ultimate test of fitness.

With this in mind I enter the war zone at my peril. Regulars had warned me that while the warm-up is no more challenging than any other, Sansome gives away nothing about what is to follow, preferring to catch his troops off-guard by making each workout as a different as possible. This time the session kicks off with press-ups and squat thrusts executed with military precision to keep in beat with the sound of Sansome's whistle.

Between each set of exercises we are asked to sprint on the spot for 15 to 30 seconds before switching from star jumps to marching to step-ups. At no point are we allowed to refill our lungs before Sansome bellows out his next order.

By the end I am not the only one whose body has surrendered to the forces of gravity. Slumped on the floor, my blackened face is running rivers down my fatigues. Comfortingly, I learn that my comrades feel the same. The general consensus is that if something hurts this much it must be worth fighting for. We are battle-scarred but not defeated. So most of us will return next week.

Verdict: "Listen you 'orrible lot, this is not the place for wimps," is Sansome's warning.

Who to Contact: For details of Bootcamp classes call LA Fitness on 02073 668080; a Bootcamp video presented by Paul Sansome is available from branches of W H Smith (£10.99).

CREW CLASS

In the beginning there were fitness bikes, then to spice them up they invented Spinning – biking classes with attitude where a team leader takes a group through their paces to the obligatory blood-pumping beat of fitness funk. Now rowing machines are getting the same treatment in the form of Crew Class.

Using the Concept II indoor rowers which are designed to stimulate the drag of water against a boat, an instructor positioned at the front of the room or gym studio leads the way in a 45 minute session of interval training, steady rowing and flat-out racing on the machines.

Classes cater for up to 15 rowers who must all keep in time with each other – anyone who pushes ahead or falls behind is easily spotted and ordered to get back on course with everyone else. As you become more experienced, though, it is possible to increase your workload while sticking to the rules.

Depending on your fitness levels you can work harder or less strenuously than other class members simply by changing the intensity of your stroke. Crew Class instructors are trained to spot poor rowing technique and give advice on how to change it to avoid the risk of back problems which are common in the sport.

For those with creaky joints, the advantage with rowing is that it is non-weight bearing, so there is less pressure on the knees and hips than if you were pounding away on a treadmill for instance. And rowing does gobble up more calories than you would use running or cycling for the same length of time.

Verdict: For those who find the rowing machine a big yawn, this is a godsend. You forget how long you have been rowing because you are working so hard to keep up. It works the upper and body simultaneously, something that many fitness classes won't do.

Who to Contact: For details of Crew Class venues call 0115 945 5522

GREAT SHAPE FOR LARGER LADIES

If your local aerobics class fails to help you work off any insecurities you have about your weight, then this could be the class for you. Here you will not see teeny bodies squeezed into tight-fitting Lycra leotards. Great Shape For Larger Ladies, launched at Danceworks gym in London two years ago, is the UK's first spin-off on an idea which took LA by storm.

Aerobics for ladies (and indeed men) of a certain size is a larger than life class that is just as likely to enhance body image and self-esteem as it is to shed pounds. Below dress size 14 and you will feel out of place at this class. Even the instructor, Kathryn Szrodecki, at Dance Works falls way outside the norm for her profession at a size 28.

But by breaking the mould in terms of what a fitness instructor should like she is also opening the doors of the gym to a group of women who otherwise may never have had the courage to enter an aerobics studio.

Women who turn up for the sessions, she says, claim to have been put off by the anti-fat attitude they detected at most gyms and most claim they would have previously been too embarrassed to don figure-hugging workout gear in public.

Classes comprise of the kind of conditioning and low impact moves found in other aerobics classes but carried out in slow motion. Heavier bodies automatically place more stress on vulnerable joints, like the knees, and Great Shape classes take this into account.

However, the benefits of taking up exercise when you are overweight are vast. For one, it means that you will reap results much more quickly than your slim-line counterparts since a 180lb body uses up considerably more energy than a 110lb body to perform the same physical tasks. A few weeks of Great Shape and you could be in, well, greater shape yourself.

Verdict: For its morale-boosting benefits it is an excellent choice if you are struggling to beat the battle of the bulge or even if your ideal size and weight leave you feeling out of place at conventional classes.

Who to Contact: Call 0207 731 7436 for details of Great Shape classes or to order a Great Shape workout video. In response to demand, classes are due to be held at gyms and health clubs nationwide this year.

REBOUNDER CIRCUITS

The Rebounder Circuit Challenge is a class in which, somewhat unusually, men outnumber women at every session. It is a variation on conventional circuit training but with the exercise stations comprising Rebounder trampets – mini-trampolines on six legs.

Running on the spot, star jumps and high knee lifts are all performed on the Rebounder which provides a much more forgiving, but equally challenging, surface than the studio floor. Sue Charlton, an instructor at the London Espree clubs, says that the big advantage is that the trampet cushions your body from impact and so protects your joints from jarring.

A class starts with some jogging on the Rebounders to warm up and get used to landing with a bounce. Technique is crucial if you want to get the most out of the 50 minutes: you should aim for middle of the bed and land with flat feet rather than on toes or heels to prevent any risk of straining your calf muscles. Stretching follows and then the class launches into the ten station circuit, five performed on the rebounder and five back on terra firma.

Rotating clockwise round the studio, everyone spends 60 seconds at each station, then rests for 45 seconds before moving on to the next exercise. Some are undoubtedly more taxing than others. Of the Rebounder stations, the Spotty Dog moves cause the most groans of discomfort; here you are required to perform scissor jumps – one foot in front of the other – while swinging your arms. Station two – running fast on the trampet, may be less jarring on the knees but it presents its own challenges.

US researchers have found that your body has to work harder to run on a springy surface like this than on a treadmill. Once everyone is back where they started, we embark on a second lap of the circuit at twice the speed. Mayhem ensues and we finish collapsed in sweat.

Verdict: Cushioned but not cushy. Physiotherapists recommend working out on a mini-trampet to protect your body. Especially beneficial if you are prone to injury.

Who to Contact: Rebounder circuits run at gyms around the country. To find out where or to purchase a rebounder call 0207 816 5353.

SPINNING

Spinning, or cycling to music, was considered an unusual concept when it first hit gyms, but now everyone's doin' it. The idea behind an indoor cycling class came from, you guessed it, the USA where professional cyclist Johnny G was searching for a way to train for the annual Los Angeles to New York bike race.

He built himself a super-sturdy, indoor bike, set it up in his garage and invited friends along to join him and relieve the tedium of hours spent pedalling alone. Reebok was so sold on the idea of the special bikes that it bought the rights to market them and Spinning was born.

Although the Spinning bikes look like any other exercise cycle, in fact they have much smoother momentum and a wide range of resistance settings so that everyone can complete a 45 minute class at their own level.

A class involves simulating a cycle ride across demanding terrain. My instructor took us up hill and down dale, asking us to sit, stand and pedal ferociously.

We also worked the upper body by pumping the handlebars to and from our chest. You will sweat, ache and moan considerably, but after three to four weeks the results of regular Spinning will be noticeable.

If you need convincing that it will get you fit too, try this: Johnny G later won the cycling race from LA to NY, covering the 3100 miles in 12 days, more than four hours ahead of the next competitor.

Verdict: If you want to lose weight and firm up quickly, then give it a spin. Not so good if you have knee problems as the pedalling action could aggravate existing aches and strains. As a calorie burner it is top notch.

US fitness experts estimate you can burn around 270 calories every 30 minutes when you Spin, more than medium paced swimming or high impact aerobics.

Who to Contact: For details of classes offering Reebok Spinning call 0113 237 1100.

STRIDES CLASS

The idea of running on a treadmill for anything longer than 20 minutes is not usually something that would inspire me to pull on my trainers. I am a huge fan of running outdoors with changing scenery to take my mind off the pain, but drumming up the enthusiasm to run indoors on a treadmill with only MTV to distract me is not easy.

Partly as a result of gym-goers bemoaning the fact that treadmills take the fun out of running, the manufacturers Powerjog came up with the format for Strides, an indoor jogging class which is to running what Spinning is to cycling. I lined up with eight other striders ranging from novice joggers to Powerjog's Andy Symonds, a former international marathon runner who helped construct the class.

Starting with a gentle five minute walk, which quickened to a jog for a further five minutes, we were taken through a range of stretching exercises for the upper body as we jogged along. Then the real work began when we were told to perform 15 bicep curls followed by 15 shoulder presses (as if raising a barbell above our heads) four times over as we ran. Later we would repeat these moves and others using weights.

We also programmed our treadmills to move a little faster for a little longer before jumping to the stationary part of the machine and performing a series of squats. It got worse. We inclined the belt of the treadmill four per cent every four minutes, sprinting at the new level until we reached a mountainous 25 per cent slope. Sweat was flying and knees were buckling around me. This kind of interval training in which periods of fast, all-out-effort are interspersed with slower, recovery work is something favoured by top athletes.

We kept it up for an hour without realising it. And then we were told we had been let off lightly. In some Strides classes, says Symonds, participants are asked to lie on their back on the still treadmill belt and perform sit-ups and press-ups. We finished with some light stretching and a jog, then walk, to cool down. So did I hit the runner's high? The answer is a resounding yes.

For the first time ever on a treadmill I felt as if I had run myself into a better mood. Next day my dead-leg syndrome reminded me how hard we had worked. And to think we had just been running on the spot.

Verdict: A good idea if you dislike or feel nervous about running alone and also if you find it difficult to summon up enthusiasm for outdoor running when it is cold and wet.

Of course, it is sociable too, so no more of the long distance runner's loneliness. It is as tough a workout as you wish to make it since you can alter the intensity and speed of your treadmill according to your level of fitness.

Who to Contact: Powerjog has details of Strides classes around the UK. For details call 0345 023038.

THE EDGE HEALTH SYSTEM

The promotional burn for this latest fitness sensation sounds promising to say the least. No more weights, aerobics classes or stair machines, now you create physical perfection out of thin air. Just sitting in the Edge Health system will help improve cardiovascular fitness say its manufacturers.

Muster up the energy to do anything remotely active in the nine foot by eight foot capsule and you are looking at increased endurance, fat and calories being gobbled up and your average workout time being sliced in half.

Top athletes have long known that training in hypoxic conditions – where less than usual levels of oxygen circulate in the air – can boost performance by making the body work harder as it acclimatises. But until now they have had to fork out thousands to travel to high altitude resorts so that they can work out in thinner air.

The oxygen-depleted Edge system, which looks like a high tech greenhouse, is said to provide all the benefits of exercising at 9000 feet above sea level without the climb. Inside, the artificial atmosphere fools your lungs into thinking they're on an alpine peak with an oxygen content of around 15 per cent compared with the normal 21 per cent at sea level.

In addition, the atmosphere is adapted to avoid the drop in barometric pressure that can cause headaches and nausea in the mountains.

A small filter extracts a pre-set amount of oxygen from the air outside and pumps the thinned-out gas into the Edge room. At New York's Crunch Fitness Club where the world's first hypoxic training room was launched two years ago, staff refer to it as the 'punishment chamber.'

I tried a 30 minute jog on a treadmill placed inside the Edge System at Holmes Place, Oxford Street in London and crawled out feeling like I had run two marathons back to back. Try it. It will take your breath away.

Verdict: Scientifically proven to be of benefit to endurance athletes who use it regularly. May also be beneficial to exercise in the Edge room for a few weeks before a skiing trip.

Who to Contact: For more information about where you can find an Edge Health System, call Hypoxico UK on 0208 325 8111.

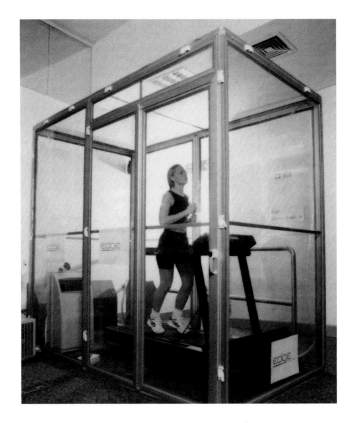

The Edge Health System

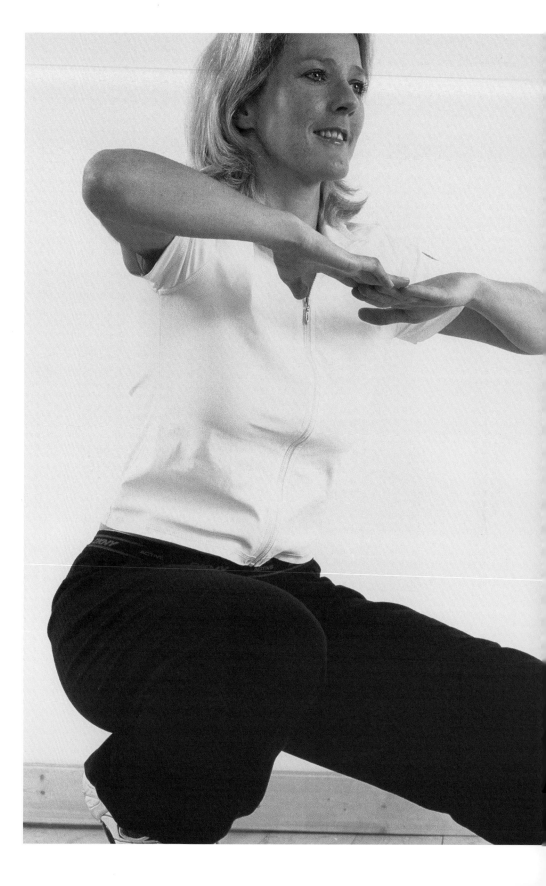

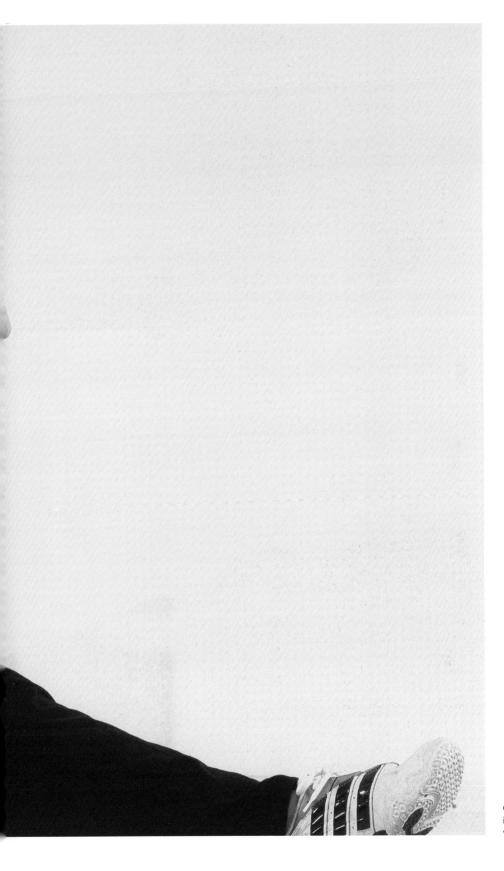

DANCE

Cossack Dancing
is absurdly hard
work

DANCE

As someone who had always required Dutch courage to shuffle onto the dance floor even at family gatherings, I was wary, to say the least, about trying any kind of organised dance class.

Yet of all the classes I have tried, it is some of these that have allowed for inhibitions to be stripped away and self expression to come to the forein whatever form. Even with the co-ordination of a plank, I have discovered that I can enjoy moving to the beat in my own fashion, so don't let lack of experience put you off.

Ethnic dance is particularly popular in gyms at the moment and classes are generally high energy but low impact. In the USA, ballet-style classes are springing up all over the place with the emphasis on increasing flexibility, strength and muscle tone rather than aerobic fitness.

For details of ballet, ballroom, line-dance, tap and modern dance contact either the British Association of Teachers of Dancing, 23 Marywood Square, Glasgow G41 2BP (0141 423 4029) or the National Association of Teachers of Dancing, 44-47 The Broadway, Thatcham, Berkshire, RG19 3HP (01635 868888).

Overall, the best place for advice when you are looking to join a dance class is the Central Council of Physical Recreation Movement and Dance Division (0207 828 3163). Write to the CCPR at Francis House, Francis Street, London, SW1P 1DE or e-mail: admin@ccpr.org.uk and they will send you details of organisations for a variety of dance forms.

AFRICAN DANCING

Big Joe Larty demonstrates to his class how to dance like a flamingo. "Jump, hop, jump and then start circling your arms faster, faster,

faster..." This we do, vainly attempting to keep in time with the beat of African drums being played by another member of Azido, the African dance troupe famed for its performances of Under African Skies, that travels the country demonstrating and teaching its art form. Together with fellow professional dancer, Mona Daniel, Larty leads us through 90 minutes of vigorous wiggling, thrusting and shaking.

There is no let-up in the action and, were it not that we were strutting our stuff in a grim, poorly ventilated room in Islington, we could well have been under African skies ourselves. It attracts a 50:50 mix of men and women, some of whom travel the breadth of Britain to attend the class on a Monday evening.

We are taught the Funky Guinea Fowl, the Towke and the Kumpo, a dance depicting the circumcision ceremony of a young boy. Granted, not your typical fitness class, but enjoyable nonetheless. The finale is a performance of what we have learned and, flamingo-flapped to the point of exhaustion, we collapse in a pool of sweat and let out a weary cheer.

Verdict: One of the few dance classes in the UK where you are guaranteed live music. Not that you even notice it being played after a few minutes of dancing. This is aerobically tough and, for first timers, choreographically challenging. But you get the hang of it when you are lured back for a second time. And you will be.

Who to Contact: African dance classes run by Azido are held throughout the year at the Canonbury Business Centre, 202 New North Road, London, N1. Weekend courses are organised every few months. For details call 0207 359 7453.

BELLY DANCING

Somewhat unfairly, belly dancing has gained a nudge, nudge, wink wink, Soho-sleaze reputation in this country but traditionally it is danced by women, for women. In the Middle East, belly dancing is a symbol of maternity and even today the female members of some tribes gather around a woman in labour and belly dance while she gives birth in the hope that their sensual swaying will somehow make the birth less of an ordeal.

In the UK, however, we remain rather more inhibited about jiggling our bare midriffs in front of others, something that Jacqueline Chapman, one of the UK's few professional belly dancers, is trying to change. Chapman is a sight to behold in her sequinned regalia as she sashays, wispy veils trailing behind her, into the studio where we are to be taught the basic rhythmic wiggling moves.

We start with some stretching and, once our muscles are warm, progress into a dance routine of sorts. Isolation of muscles is the key to mastering the art we are told, and the head, neck and chest should be kept still but in relaxed alignment with the body. But it takes practice before the act of gyrating your previously immobile midriff resembles anything like a dance. However, when you have grasped the idea that it requires complete abandonment of self-consciousness, you are half way there.

Also Try

There cannot be many fitness classes where an expanding waistline is praised and rotund stomachs openly flaunted, but BELLY BABIES, also taught by Jacqueline Chapman, is one. In what is undoubtedly the country's most unusual ante-and post-natal exercise course, Chapman teaches belly dancing to women who want to stay in shape during pregnancy.

A trained nurse, she came up with the idea after wiggling her way through her own four pregnancies and retaining her feminine curves. Regular dancing means blood supply to the abdominal area is boosted and, when the pelvic floor muscles are exercised, common gynaecological problems related to pregnancy – stress incontinence and even constipation – are markedly reduced.

Verdict: Belly dancing is not a great aerobic workout, but for toning, mobility and improving self-confidence, it takes some beating. Suitable for most ages and all levels of fitness. Most beginners arrive in leggings and baggy t-shirts. By week three they are adorned in glittery accessories, tassels and veils. A great excuse to dress up.

Who to Contact: For details of Belly Dancing classes, Belly Babies or individual tuition by Jacqueline Chapman send an SAE to Belly Dancing, 585 Watford Way, Mill Hill, London, NW7 3JG; send an SAE to The Dance Development officer, Central Council for Physical Recreation, Francis House, Francis Street, London, SW1P 1DE for other classes.

BREAK DANCING

It had to happen. With the current revival of all things Eighties, Break Dancing was bound to make a comeback sooner or later. Life in that decade was not complete without the dance form that brought us Michael Jackson's moonwalk and the headspin. Committed break dancers or b-boyers, as they are now known, will tell you that it never really disappeared – it just took a backward flip in the popularity stakes.

However, this time around it has also been given the green light by those who dictate what is good for us. The Health Education Authority (HEA) has backed it as a means of getting into shape – provided you don't try any of the moves which involve balancing on your head. Bad news those. Presumably I was in the throes of mid-adolescent turmoil when the first craze hit and was far too self-conscious to risk my limbs letting me down in public because I never got around to break dancing in the 1980s. So it is as a complete novice that I join the Magic Circle b-boyers to learn the tricks of the trade.

Once we get started it becomes obvious that acquiring the skills to perform an impromptu, traffic-stopping display of break dancing could involve a lengthier process of tuition than we first thought. Hang loose and go with the flow is the general theme of things, but even the apparently simple moves – such as sending an imaginary shock-wave from one outstretched arm, through my torso, to the other – looks nothing like a dance move when I try it.

After an hour of effort I am closer to the mark, kicking and jerking with some style. At 13, I would have walked through walls to develop such skills. Now I know I am far too long in the tooth to care whether anyone knows if I can breakdance and I moonwalk my way back to my car.

Verdict: Tough on the muscles and, provided you do it continuously for 20 minutes or longer, a good aerobic workout. A lot of the moves are performed at ground level and involve balancing on one limb for several seconds which improves strength. But, whichever way you look at it, age is a limiting factor.

Who to Contact: Send an SAE to Health Education Authority/Active for Life, Trevelyan House, 30 Great Peter Street, London, SW1P 2HW for information about break dancing; send an SAE to The Dance Development officer, Central Council for Physical Recreation, Francis House, Francis Street, London, SW1P 1DE for details of dance workshops.

COSSACK DANCING

Turning up for a session with the Mazeppa Cossack dancers, the first professional group of its kind outside the Ukraine, I was unsure what to expect. I knew it might involve lots of crouching down and kicking my legs from beneath me. I also knew the technique was tricky to grasp because I tried it once at a party. But that was my sum knowledge of this energetic dance form. Perhaps, then, the warm up routine should have provided sufficient warning that my muscles were in for a difficult ride.

Led by the dancer Dmitz Torkoniak, I have to jog, stretch extensively and then perform short sprints to loosen up my legs. Maybe it is the odd physical challenge of Cossack dancing that gives it appeal. The Central Council of Physical recreation says that an increasing number of more unusual dance forms are gaining in popularity among those who have had their fill of the treadmill.

The traditions of Cossack dancing are remarkable. During the war when Ukrainian immigrants settled in the UK, Canada and Australia social clubs were established so that the spirit of the national dance might live on. I started with an exercise which involved me jumping in the air and landing with one leg bent and the other stretched out to the side in a lunge position. I realised why I had been told to wear loose, unrestrictive clothing.

Anything else would seriously have hindered my chances of walking out of the room the same way I had walked in. Other moves, thankfully, require the assistance of a partner which reduces the workload a little. I tried the Cobbler – legs bent, arms folded in front of me in classic Cossack pose – but didn't impress the others. Or myself, for that matter.

Verdict: This is absurdly hard work. Take me back to the gym.

Who to Contact: For information about traditional dance classes, including Cossacks, in your area, send an SAE to: Dance Development Officer, Central Council for Physical Recreation, Francis House, Francis Street, London, SW1P 1DE.

DISCO 2000

You know you are edging ever closer towards shaking off these mortal coils when the decade through which you attended school becomes cool once more in a retro way. Disco 2000, as its name suggests, is a 45 minute workout inspired by Seventies dance movies and music. It is the brainchild of award winning fitness instructor Alex Rees and leading choreographer Andy Roberts who had long suspected that boogieing antics would be an effective aerobic workout and devised this routine to the music of the Jacksons, the Bee Gees, Odyssey and the rest.

The session starts in much the same way as any other with some marching, stepping and stretching performed to the softer 'lurve' songs of the decade. Ten minutes into the class and the real work starts.

We are taught a variety of dance techniques from the Funky Chicken (hands on hips, arms flapping to the side) to the Travolta (sultry look, one hand on hip, one arm swooping in front of you). Requires total concentration and there were arms and legs akimbo as we struggled to get it right. By the end Rees says we gave a performance to Night Fever that did us justice. Hmmm.

Verdict: Disco dancing works the aerobic system much harder than many other forms of exercise because it requires vigorous movements all the time.

Plenty of crouching and swooping-to-the-floor means the legs work hard too.

On average you will burn as many calories (around 365 for a 10st woman) doing this for one hour as you would cycling ten miles in the same time.

Who to Contact: The Disco 2000 workout will be introduced to gyms and health clubs throughout 2000. For more information or to order a Disco 2000 workout video (£12.50), call : 0208 744 9443.

SALSA

That the Latin Americans are passionate souls becomes apparent the moment you try salsa dancing for yourself. Even for those who struggle to exhibit any sensuality on a disco floor, a certain degree of sexiness is guaranteed when you salsa.

Part of the sizzle comes from the music, but the steps themselves – including the shimmy, swivel and exotic head throw – can trigger hormonal rumblings between partners. An hour or so after being introduced to my partner, who was unknown to me before my lesson and who made such a swift exit afterwards that I never got to know his name, I was wiggling, snake-hipped style around him as if we were intimately acquainted.

The average beginner's class lasts one hour and runs for six weeks by which time you should have perfected the basic steps. Don't think you will get an easy ride – this is vigorous and demanding enough to leave you dripping with sweat when you crawl off the dance floor at the end. It is recommended that you bring your partner, lest they begin to suspect you are falling for the dancer, not the dance.

Verdict: Experts agree that Salsa, being one of the more energetic forms of dance, is an excellent work out, typically raising the heart rate to around 70 per cent of its maximum and helping to burn as many calories as you would jogging at a slow pace. Also great for strengthening the calf muscles and those in the thigh and buttocks.

Who to Contact: For details of classes in your area, send an A4 SAE to British Dance Council, Terpsichore House, 240 Merton Road, London, SW19 1EQ.

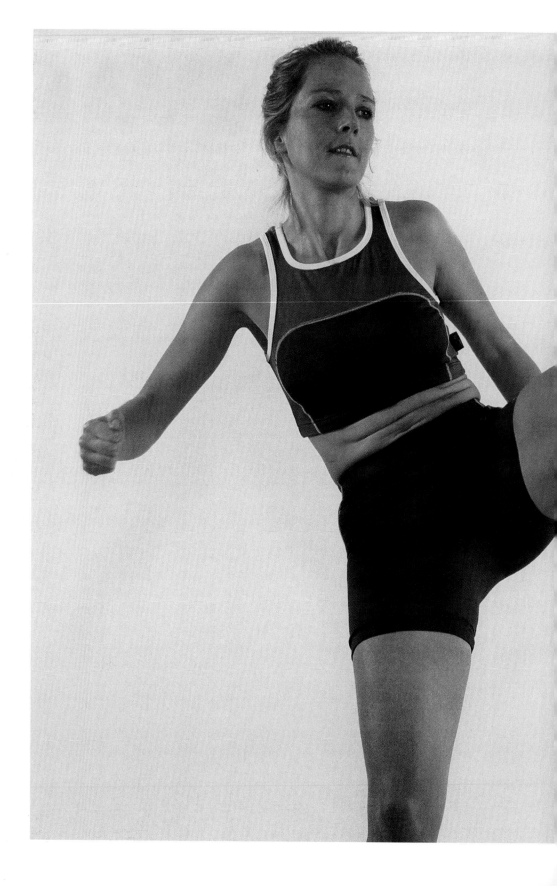

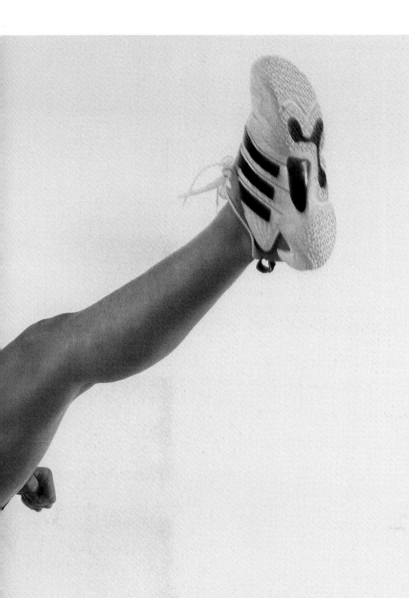

MARTIAL ARTS

Kick Boxing
just like
Sporty Spice

MARTIAL ARTS

If you have been put off trying a martial art due to lingering visions of Bruce Lee and his Kung-fu kicks or a fear of being slam-dunked over the shoulder of a mean-eyed man in a white linen suit, then maybe you should take a fresh look at what is on offer.

Thanks largely to the celebrity endorsement of classes like Billy Blanks' Tae Bo in Los Angeles, martial-art inspired fitness is booming at the moment on both sides of the Atlantic.

Many classes on offer in gyms present diluted versions of a traditional art form and the likes of combat training, cardio combat and others are a mix of kicks and conventional aerobic routines. They are an ideal place to start if you are completely new to the idea of fighting your way to fitness.

Most martial arts include some kicking and a lot of lower body work which make them an excellent way to strengthen the legs. And considering it takes nine times the energy to produce a strong high-kick as it does to punch, then it is hardly surprising that you can burn around 700 calories in one 45 minute class. Flexibility, strength and a good aerobic conditioning workout make it one of the best all-round workouts on offer.

If you do opt for a conventional martial art, then there are added spiritual benefits, especially if you choose something like T'ai Chi. Unlike the gym-based classes, martial arts are traditionally done in silence which supposedly helps to build inner focus and calm.

A study in the journal of Sports Behaviour showed that people who regularly take part in a martial art reported feeling calmer, less stressed and more focussed in other areas of their lives.

CAPOEIRA

The Junga is the basic move of Capoeira. It appears effortless. Side step to the right, then the left and swing your arms correspondingly. Yet the rules of this Brazilian martial art form mean that you must do it within the confines of a chalk-drawn circle on the gym floor while keeping to the beat of a an odd-looking one-stringed instrument called the Berimbau.

Worse, you must do it in full view of your classmates who chant and cheer as you to try to out-jinga-swing an opponent. Capoeira transpired to be a curious combination of elegant dance moves, powerful high kicks and, by some, a display of daunting acrobatic moves.

This martial art is steeped in tradition. Back in the 18th century, millions of Africans were taken as slaves to Brazil where their repressive masters decreed fighting a crime punishable by the loss of a hand. So the slaves developed a form of martial combat disguised as a dance to deter suspicion.

In Brazil it remains massively popular as a competitive sport, but in trendy US gyms it is rapidly usurping more conventional martial arts like Tae Kwon Do. It requires you to do more than bust a gut in the name of fitness. It is as mentally challenging as it is physical.

Our instructor, Master Ousado, a native Brazilian, first takes us through the basic movements which mostly involve crouching down at floor level and pivoting on either one hand or a foot. The aim, says Ousado, is to appear graceful under pressure and to make it look as if we are moving fluidly even when it seems to us that we are just jerking from one position to the next. The entire class ran for one-and-a-half exhausting hours and at the end we were summoned to sit around the edge of the circle and display what we have learned in a mock battle with a partner.

Capoeira is a game of wits and the idea is not to out-muscle the opposition but to cunningly out-fox him. I didn't last long, but not to worry, says Ousado, as progress is swift. I left the room elated but weary.

Verdict: It can be off-putting to see experienced Capoeirists cartwheeling around the room in your first session, but persevere and your increased flexibility, speed, balance and agility will astound you. But you will ache for days when you first start.

Who to Contact: For more information contact the London School of Capoeira on 0207 2812020; for details of Capoeira and other martial arts classes call the Amateur Martial Arts Association on 0207 837 4406.

KARATE

The English translation of the Japanese word Karate means 'empty hand,' a reference to the fact that this teaches you how to fight unarmed. Karate is a form of self-defence which relies on tremendous power from the legs and abdominal muscles to carry out the moves. Most classes will last over an hour and incorporate a full range of fitness disciplines from stretching to punching and kicking and, once you have mastered the basics, some sparring with a partner.

Karate is a competitive sport and not one that you will generally find run as a fitness class in trendy gyms. However beginners are welcomed to Karate clubs, so check with the governing bodies for the nearest to you. If you like it, you will be encouraged to work your way through the graded belt system.

Verdict: You do not have to be physically strong to take up Karate although your overall strength to weight ratio will increase if you keep it up, leaving you with more toned muscle all over. The emphasis is on speedy footwork and quick reactions, so agility, balance and co-ordination will also improve.

Who to Contact: English Karate on 01225 834008 (www.ekgb.org.uk); Karate Union of Great Britain on 0151 652 1208 or the Amateur Martial Arts Association on 0207 837 4406

KENDO

If you like the idea of a real fight, then Kendo could be the sport for you.

This Japanese martial art was devised by Samurai Warriors thousands of years ago. In those days real swords were used in the battle, but today bamboo replacements make do. Still, it is tremendous swashbuckling fun and for 90 minutes or longer you will learn sword and sparring skills with a partner.

The aim is to strike your opponent in target areas including points on the body and head. You rarely get hit hard. Well, OK, maybe the odd bruise...

Verdict: Since you are fully armed with protective gear provided by the Kendo clubs for beginners (which can weigh up to 24lbs) and a mock sword, simply moving around will require effort. Strength in the forearms, aerobic fitness, reaction times and mental awareness will also improve with regular Kendo sessions.

Who to Contact: British Kendo Association on 01843 592472.

KICK BOXING

Caprice, Sporty Spice, Mel C and hordes of Hollywood babes count this as their favourite martial art. Kick Boxing is a mix of Kung-fu and Karate that became a sport in its own right in the 1950s in the US and made its way over here in the 1970s. Unlike other martial arts classes, you generally need to be kitted out in gloves – although person to person contact is not obligatory, you will be required to hit at pads.

Footwork skills, kicking and punching are all taught. Classes generally last 50 minutes to an hour, starting with a dynamic warm up and intense stretching.

Verdict: Be prepared to work hard and sweat buckets. The results, however, will be improved muscle definition, especially in the arms, bottom and thighs, as well as better flexibility. Kick Boxing is a good cardiovascular workout too.

Who to Contact: The Contact Sports Union on 0121 242 1356 or the National College of Karate on 0207 278 5608.

TAE BO

Tae-what? You may well ask. In fact, this is one of Hollywood's hottest classes. Led by fitness guru Billy Blanks, seven times world Karate champion and a black belt in Tae Kwon Do, the 150 devotees who regularly queue to get into his class in Sherman Oaks, downtown LA, include Goldie Hawn, Carmen Electra, Brooke Shields and Sugar Ray Leonard. Blanks then leads them through his unique one-hour hybrid of activity which comprises Tae Kwon Do, hip-hop dancing and boxing steps.

The benefits, claim Tae Bo converts, are that, unlike traditional martial arts sessions in which the emphasis is on repeating techniques slowly and methodically until you get them right, in this class you repeat kick punches in quick succession and a high number of repetitions to get the fat-burning effects.

And by all accounts, it works – the US magazine, Muscle and Fitness, recently rated Tae Bo as the highest calorie-burning workout around, estimating that when you become proficient at the kicks you can burn 800 calories an hour.

Now you can try Tae Bo over here. In all but name that is. Since

Blank's feathers have been ruffled of late by those intent on cashing in on his success, the class must be called something different in the UK. So we have the likes of Tai Bo, Tae Bow and Fighting Fit. Anne Marie Millard, martial arts expert and a Fighting Fit instructor, tells me that regular sessions will leave me with biceps like tennis balls and overall upper and lower body strength like I have never known.

We jog and side step for ten minutes before Millard takes us through the moves, teaching us how to kick at a Tae Kwon Do paddle from different angles and punch wearing a pair of bag gloves. The session lasts an hour and we cool down with some light stretches.

Verdict: You will feel stiff the next day after high-kicking and punching for at least 45 minutes. Classes vary considerably in the UK.

However find a good one, as a calorie burner and aerobic fitness booster, it is one of the best. The American Council on exercise recently reported that the average combat-style class will burn 450 calories.

Who to Contact: Gyms around the UK are now holding their own version, including Holmes Place clubs' Thai-Bo (call 0207 374 0091); for details of Fighting Fit, call 0208 374 6087 or send an SAE to Fighting Fit, 99 Middle Lane, Crouch end, London, N8 8NX.

T'AI CHI

This ancient art form has been described as an internal Kung-fu; a means of banishing your inner beasts and replacing them with positive inner energies.

Its philosophy suggests that you stand like a mountain and flow like a river to attain this spiritual calm. As a result, doing T'ai Chi moves in front of the TV or while wearing a set of head phones is a no-no. It was created originally by a Chinese monk in the 13th century and is based on the Taoist beliefs that internal forces of yin and yang must be balanced if we are to remain healthy in body and mind. Through focusing on the four principles of the martial art – posture, internal energy, chi (life energy) and mind – you will learn how to replace negative forces with positive ones.

Movements are slow and controlled. Admittedly you will gain virtually nothing when it comes to aerobic fitness and it features pretty low on the calorie and fat burning scales too. Still, some moves do help to improve strength (if you are standing on one leg for example) and you will definitely increase flexibility and balance.

But forget sweating. The main advantage has to be that a session of T'ai Chi will set you up mentally for the day ahead. In fact, proponents recommend beating the morning rush of joggers to the local park where you can be at one with yourself and meditate in a relatively peaceful environment. Don't be phased by onlookers walking their dogs who stare, eyes narrowed, as you work at rebalancing your chi.

This really works.

Verdict: S-l-o-w-l-y does it. If you want to shrink the size of your derriere, this is not the place to do it.

Who to Contact: The T'ai Chi Centre on 0207 486 9957.

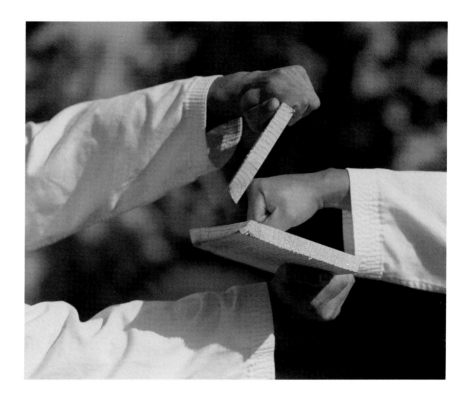

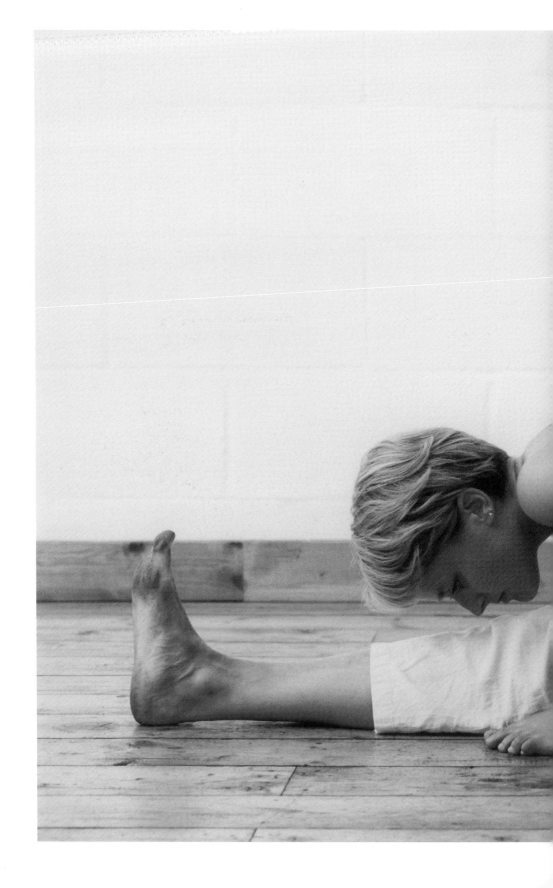

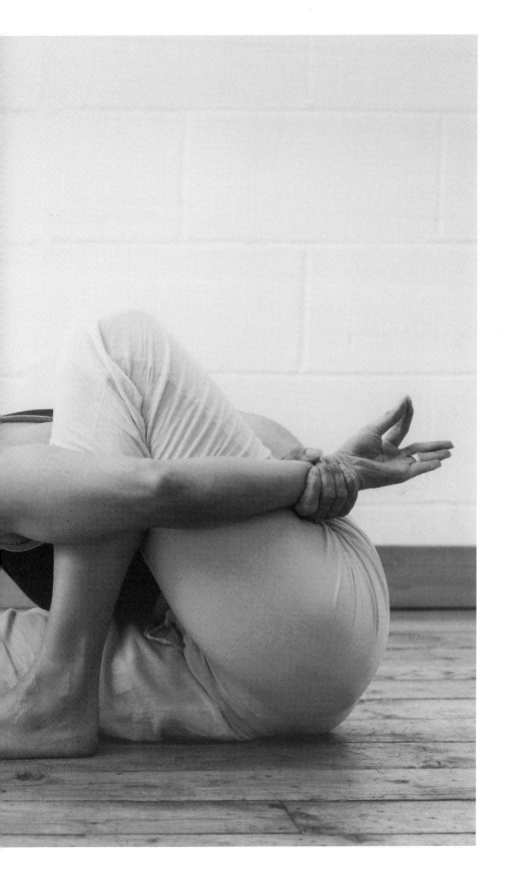

MIND & BODY

Yoga: finally
got a new
image

MIND & BODY

Last year I interviewed Gin Miller, the American fitness guru who invented the Step Reebok phenomenon in the 1980s after stepping up and down on a milk crate in her back garden and thinking, hey, this is a great way to keep in shape. She sold the idea to Reebok and what followed was nothing short of a step aerobics craze that endures to this day – a low impact, high energy class with the primary aim of reducing the size of those body parts we love to hate.

But over the years Miller admitted to having a niggling doubt that her fitness sensation really was the ultimate answer to all-round fitness. What was missing, she said, was any attention to the development of the spirit as people in their thousands clambered on and off their specially-constructed plastic boxes in the name of acquiring a waistline. Hence, towards the end of the Nineties, she became one of the fitness industry's most vocal proponents for what is almost definitely to become the exercise revolution of this Millennium.

Mind-body fitness aims to address the spirit, soul and muscles in one session. It comes in many different guises and some forms are far more effective than others, just as some minds and bodies will be far better suited to one class than another. Yet the common theme is that you need to attain an inner balance to attain an outer one and in order to feel content with the way you look, you must be content with the way you feel inside.

CHI-BALL

The first thing that will strike you about a Chi-Ball class is not the unique combination of exercises drawn from yoga, Pilates and other mind-body classes, but the overwhelmingly sweet scent that fills the room when you walk in. Chi-Balls, six-inch diameter rubber balls, are dowsed with different aromatherapy oils, each billed to have a specific effect on your mood. For stress magnets, lavender balls are the order of the day as the scent will soothe and relax, while those with low self-esteem should select an orange scented ball to boost self-confidence.

The theme of the class, which is Australian by design, is part Chinese medicine and part postural fitness. According to practitioners of Chinese medicine, chi is the life force which flows freely through our bodies when we are well but becomes blocked when we are overworked, overtired and ill. In a Chi-Ball class, participants first learn to breathe deeply enough to affect the chi and ensure that oxygen reaches the vital organs.

Exercises are mainly gentle and flowing – there is no aerobic charging around – with the ball being held in position to help control stability and alignment. A significant section of the class is devoted to lengthening the spine through a range of stretching and strengthening moves and towards the end, the entire body unwinds and relaxes through Feldenkrais exercises. This unusual postural technique, which is rapidly gaining popularity in its own right at health clubs and gyms around the UK, is based on the natural and uninhibited movements of children who crawl and manoeuvre themselves in the most practical and efficient ways.

At the end of the class it is considered a positive sign if you are hot and bothered in spite of a minimum level of vigorous movement. It is believed that bodily heat is a sign that chi is moving freely through the body. You may also discover that headaches, minor tummy pains and other niggles will disappear after just one hour-long class.

Verdict: A perfect end to a stressful day. Do not expect to grind and burn, but to unwind gradually and emerge feeling fully stretched out both spiritually and physically. Many of the Pilates and yoga movements are beneficial for posture and alignment.

Who to Contact: Chi-Ball classes are being introduced at gyms and health clubs around the country including Holmes Place and the David Lloyd Clubs. Chi Ball videos are also available, complete with a ball. Call 01225 700059 for details.

CHUA KA

Chua Ka, a do-it yourself massage therapy, was invented in the 1960s by US psychologist, Oscar Ichazo, who believes that different parts of the body store specific fears and that regular head-to-toe massage can not only make us more supple and less inclined to physical strain, but will also flush out the toxins that trigger a whole range of negative emotions. It uses such varied tools as a cooking spatula, bicarbonate of soda and liver salts.

According to the principles of Chua Ka, each area of the body is also a zone of karma that will accumulate stress to a greater or lesser extent depending on what has been causing us strife most recently. Tension in the feet, for instance, is considered an indication that you are suffering from low self-esteem and are afraid 'to be yourself'; a stiff neck could mean that you are guilty, a sore chin that you feel inferior and so on. As might be expected of something which claims to help ease such deep-rooted feelings, Chua Ka requires you to do more than just glide your hands over the surface of your skin with sweet-scented oils. Instead, using your fingers, and occasionally a Ka stick (or wooden spatula), as massage tools, you work at a much deeper level.

Starting at the feet, we are shown how to use our fingers to 'chisel' into muscles, stopping just before the point of pain. We work through the body in zones. On larger areas, such as the thigh and calf muscles, we apply the same sort of pressure with the spatula. Our instructor explains how toxic deposits that cause the skin to stick to the muscles like glue and that massaging the skin helps to cleanse the area. Amid murmurs of approval she also tells us that it is a wonderful way to get rid of cellulite. It is because of all this toxic release that we need to stay well-hydrated and why we are advised to keep sipping at a glass of water mixed with liver salts – a natural internal cleanser. It is also a good idea, we are told, to add a packet of bicarbonate of soda to our bath water after a self-massage session to help get rid of any toxins on the skin's surface.

Verdict: Ideal pampering for anyone who exercises regularly. More strenuous than it sounds.

Who to Contact: For details, send an SAE to MetaFitness, Squire's Hill House, Tilford, Surrey, GU10 2AD (01252 782661).

SESH (Egyptian Stretching)

As I sit red faced and grimacing with my back straight and fingers digging into the floor beside me, a 14st man uses his entire body weight to pin my knees to the ground. After holding the position for what seems like an eternity I am told to give him my right leg which he hoists up to his shoulder so that my foot is more or less level with the top of his head.

Given that neither of my legs is generally required to scale such heights I am pretty chuffed just to see it up there, but my teacher in this Sesh class is not as easily impressed and starts inching my straightened limb towards my ear. While I am being contorted, he explains that these movements form some of the most basic (basic!) postures of Sesh, an ancient Egyptian training regime that aims to push back the boundaries of physical and mental inhibition.

The idea is that with a little practice and a certain amount of willpower we can all bend and shape ourselves like this for the benefit of our health. Sesh incorporates four forms of flexibility in each posture – yoga, isometric or flex and relax stretches and passive moves where you hold the muscles in one position for a certain time. A few deep breathing exercises are followed by, and I kid you not, a

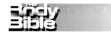

simultaneous cracking of joints by everyone in the room. This is to prepare us for the foot-flexing movements which follow and at which I fail miserably. My inability to isolate my big toes and move them clockwise while keeping my other toes still is, apparently, a sign that my body is one big stress magnet. Moving on from the feet we progress into a series of dynamic stretches, such as grasping the feet with my hands, then straightening my legs while balancing on my bottom for a count of 30. Then there are the one-handed push-ups.

Oh no, Sesh is not a sloucher's option. For 48 hours afterwards I cursed the fool who invented stairs. And to think I had expected something like yoga.

Verdict: Strengthens both the mind and the body. If you can get through this, anything else is a breeze.

Who to Contact: For more information about Sesh, write to The Ancient Egyptian Cultural Centre, PO Box 2386 London, W1A 2RF.

THE LAVENDER WORKOUT

Classes that afford equal attention to mind and body are not new. Yoga and the like have been around for thousands of years. But this is perhaps the only gym class I have come across which devotes more time to the old grey matter than to your muscles. In the Lavender Workout, the emphasis is on, well, lying down. You lie down when you enter the room and don't get up again until it's time to leave and the Bums Tums and Thighs crowd are hammering on the studio door to get in.

Lavender scent wafts from incense burners dotted around the floor and our instructor, Paul Sansome, entertains us with humourous stories "to clear the air of subconscious confrontational energy" for the first few minutes. Next we were taken through a process of physical relaxation in which each body part was tensed and then allowed to unwind, starting at the feet and working up to the head. This took 15 minutes or so by which time I was drifting into sleepy consciousness. Sansome then took us on a journey to open up our senses, a technique known as visualisation and something that is regularly practised by elite athletes in preparation for competition. We were told to imagine lying on the deck of a yacht, listening to the gentle lapping of waves, feeling the warmth of the sun. Eventually we are counted back up to reality again only to find that it was raining outside. Drat.

Verdict: A welcome relief from muscular and mental stress. Mid-day is the most popular time for the class.

Who to Contact: LA Fitness on 0207 366 8080.

WANDERING

This could only hail from America where, on the various occasions I have visited, it strikes me that walking in any form is an activity that is frowned upon by the masses. So, someone took the concept of a good old-fashioned stroll and marketed it as 'Wandering,' the latest way to hoist your butt and free your mind of tension. To wander is to explore your surroundings with head held high as opposed to scurrying along oblivious to your surroundings.

Focus on taking deep breaths and concentrate on the present not the past or what might happen in the next 24 hours, say enthusiasts. In fact, there are no rules as such but regular wanderers advocate following your nose rather than a pre-set route and relax as you stroll. Don't be ruled by your watch either, but do aim to be out for 20 minutes.

Of course, the real attraction to wandering is that it removes some of the rigidity we have become used to at gyms. The time is yours and you are in sole control of how much effort you do (or don't) put in.

Still, it was never going to be long before the fitness industry got wind of the fact that plain old walking is what we like doing most to burn off the calories and in the UK there are now wandering classes of sorts. Walk Reebok is a group fitness session in which you stroll or power walk depending on your objectives, under the watchful eye of an instructor. This I have tried with instructor Peter Wilmott who led me and a tribe over the hillocks and footpaths surrounding a gym in west London Industrial Estate. Sure, I sweated by the end and probably burned off some flab. But it didn't benefit my psyche half as much as a meandering around my local park. So here's to wandering, the oldest form of exercise known to man. Yet, in my humble opinion, still the best.

Verdict: Versatile of course. And strolling along at 3mph will also burn 70 calories in 20 minutes. Walk up a slight incline and you will use a third more calories.

Who to Contact: For details about Walk Reebok classes call 0113 237 1100.

YOGA

Yoga has finally shaken off its wholesome, hippy image and now it is estimated that 300,000 of us flock regularly, mat in hand, to contort ourselves like pretzels in the name of inner and outer contentment. These days, it is so popular that deciding on the yoga class to suit is no mean feat in itself. There are literally hundreds of variations to choose from.

Most classes in the west fall under the umbrella title of Hatha yoga which simply means they involve physical, rather than solely meditative, activity. Whatever banner the class falls under – be it power yoga, Iyengar or Bikram – its basic structure will probably have derived from the same set of postures or asanas as any other. There are thousands of asanas, although most classes dip into a bank of about 150, and they are known to benefit nerves, vital organs, glands and joints as well as muscles.

Studies in the US have shown that regular yoga can help lower the risk of diabetes and decrease blood pressure. The breathing techniques, which distinguish yoga from other stretching classes are what will give you the sense of mental and physical togetherness once you get the hang of things.

Flexibility, co-ordination and your ability to handle stress will also improve after a few months of doing yoga regularly. As a basic guide, Ashtanga yoga is the most physically demanding and the best for losing weight, Lyengar focuses on improving posture and physical alignment, Bikram is held in a room heated to 107 degrees and is ideal for people suffering mild, persistent back pain and Jnana is recommended for those wanting to embark on the philosophical path to spirituality.

Sivananda Yoga

It is largely thanks to the likes of Madonna, a yoga enthusiast who chants in Sanskrit on her best-selling Ray of Light album, and other celebrity chanters – Christy Turlington, Sarah Jessica Parker and designer Donna Karan, all regulars at New York's hip Jivamutki Yoga Centre – that this previously unpopular form of the yoga suddenly finds itself plunged into the spotlight. Add to this the fact that, in a study at the Preventative Medicine Research Centre in California, it was shown that yoga combined with chanting helped patients with heart disease control their stress levels and it is little wonder that it is attracting those who fed up with the race to stay on life's treadmill are taking it up in their thousands.

Sivananda differs from other yoga classes in that the repetition of postures, or asanas, leaves you sweating but they are interspersed with calmer periods of mantra therapy. The class I joined at the Holmes Place Barbican club in London started with the lighting of incense burners and chanting the verses of a Sanskrit prayer. Collectively we repeated a mantra and then sat in silence to rid our minds of stressful thoughts.

The class starts with some slow stretches, known as Sun poses, and is followed by repetitions of some of the classical yoga poses. For those who haven't tried supporting themselves with the palms of their hands and tips of their toes indefinitely before, then these types of moves are demanding enough in themselves. Yoga relies entirely on the body's own weight to provide resistance and improve overall strength and judging by the extent to which I wobbled my way through the various postures, it is something I should work at improving.

Some yoga devotees claim it is a spiritual life-saver, crowning it in religious glory. But, of course, while it addresses the needs of both body and mind more efficiently and effectively than most, it remains a run-of-the-mill fitness class. So don't be fooled on that score. Like other forms of yoga, Sivananda can be an effective means of re-evaluating life because it provides you with a snatched 90 minutes to yourself. Which, if we are to be as stressed out in this Millennium as we were in the last, can only be a good thing.

Verdict: In the USA, where this class is already established in many gyms, it has a reputation for causing people to well up with emotion. The reason for this, says Sivananda instructor Anton Michael Rocke, is that it presents you with time for your own thoughts and a period of calm in which to re-acquaint yourself with your personal space. Even if all this sounds like spiritual mumbo jumbo, it is worth a try – it might work.

Who to Contact: For details of Sivananda classes in your area, contact the Sivananda Yoga Centre, 51 Felsham Road, London, SW15 1AZ (0208 780 0160).

Tantric Yoga

It is worthwhile remembering that whichever form of yoga you choose, it remains a word loaded with a hundred innuendos as I discovered when I announced I was hooked on it to a group of friends. Hmmm. Eyes narrowed in suspicion as in the dark recesses of their minds they recalled tales of how yoga can also enhance your sex life. Unfortunately I can vouch that, apart from becoming a little more limber in bed, this is not generally the case and even the yogis in India who can retain semen do so only after decades of practice.

Now, the ancient practice of Tantric yoga, of course, is an altogether different story. A friend of mine was once dispatched to cover a Tantric yoga workshop, one of many held over weekends around the country. His intention, he says, was to find out whether he really would be able to redefine his spiritual and sexual self, as had been claimed in the brochure and to record his experiences for the benefit of his readers.

Although the prospect of 48 hours of total sexual abandonment with a group of strangers did, I feel, help sway his decision. He returned with his account of how a married couple in their fifties taught the importance of erotic touch, feathers and fingers tickling the back, and how the group was advised to try regular chanting and meditation to fire up their sexual energies. On reflection, my friend was not convinced that he had managed to centre his being but was satisfied to leave with a revitalised appetite for life, love and sex. Oh, and yoga of course.

Who to Contact: For a list of qualified instructors in your area, send an SAE to British Wheel of Yoga, 1 Hamilton Place, Boston Road, Sleaford, Lincolnshire, NG34 7ES (01529 306 851). For classes that focus on meditation techniques, send an SAE to the Sivananda Yoga Vedanta Centre, 51 Felsham Road, London, SW15 1AZ (0208 780 0160); for Tantric yoga workshops send an SAE to SkyDancing UK, 47 Maple Road, Horfield, Bristol, BS7 8RE.

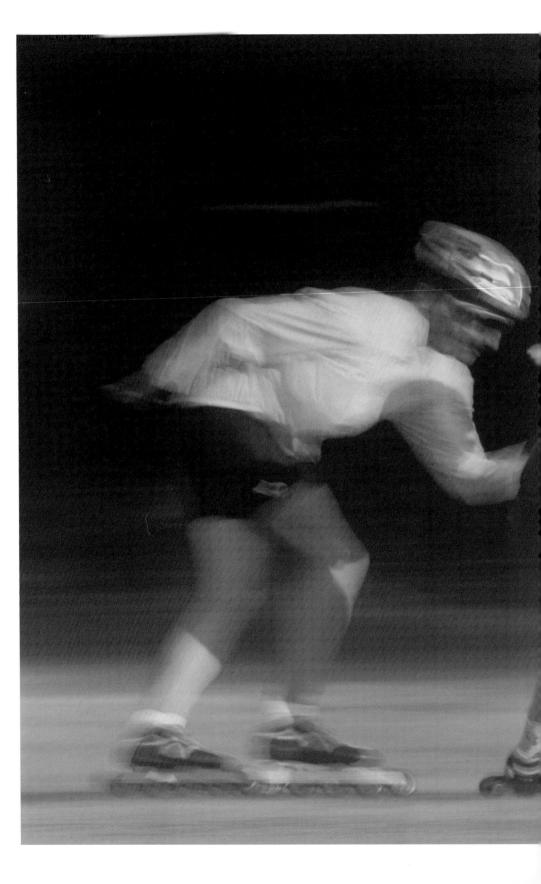

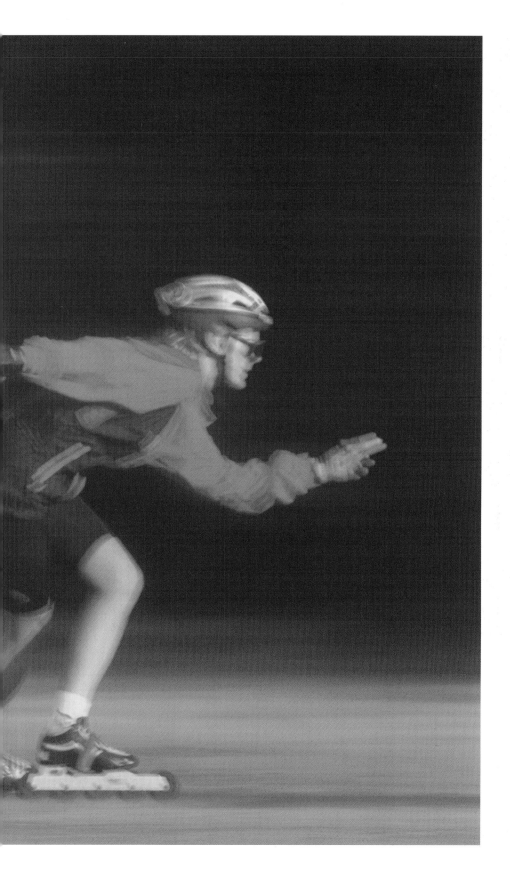

In-Line
Skating:
pedestrians
beware!

OUTDOORS

During the summer of 1999, the number of celebrities – everyone from Meg Ryan to Alanis Morisette by all accounts – who were abandoning the stuffy gym in favour of the fresh air outside inspired the Express newspaper to use the headline 'Outdoors is the New Indoors.' The great outdoors, it seems, really is the gym of the new Millennium.

Exercising outdoors need not necessarily involve organised games or activities. Anything goes, as long as you are working up a sweat. Indeed, a recent survey by US toy manufacturers revealed that adults are buying 20 per cent more outdoor toys, like kites, for their own use than they were two years ago. A sign, perhaps, that adults are finally coming round to the idea that exercising needn't be as tiresome as we so often make it and that it can even be a form of escapism from the intense world of adulthood. A strenuous game of Frisbee with an inept partner who forces you to run huge distances to catch it will amount to a good aerobic workout and will help you burn around 150 calories in 15 minutes. Call it satisfying your inner child, call it a refusal to grow up, but enjoy throwing that Frisbee.

Wearing the right clothing has a huge impact on the enjoyment you will gain from any outdoor activity. Opt for thin layers of specially designed sports fabrics for more strenuous sports and shoes with ample support around the ankle to cope with uneven terrain. For park games wear loose, comfortable clothing that allows a full range of movement.

While the Hollywood glitterati enthuse about how bonding with Mother Nature by exercising outside provides them with a unique environment in which to pursue physical and spiritual enhancement, for the rest of us the pulling power of the local park is rather more practical, of course. Unlike a hefty gym subscription, this is free...

ADVENTURE RACING

Take a triathlon, throw in mud, a kayak, some rocky and undulating terrain. What you have are the ingredients for an adventure race, the UK's latest sport import from the States. Adventure racing made it big time over here in 1999 with, among other trials of endurance and spirit, the launch of the Hi-Tec series of races in which I competed. What really distinguishes the adventure race from a regular triathlon is not merely the distance or range of activities you are required to complete, but the fact that you must do so as part of a team and must stick with the other members for the entire absurd journey.

In most cases, if you don't cross the finish line together you will not even merit an official finishing time. Let alone a burial. Still, it appears there are plenty of gluttons for this sort of punishment. The first Hi-Tec event held at Bewl Water in Kent was fully subscribed with 750 competitors weeks before it was due to take place. The one-day event takes anything from two to eight hours to complete depending on how competently your team tackles the kayaking, running, mountain biking and 'mystery' challenges thrown in for good measure. As the obligatory female member of a three-strong squad that took part in the event I am to this day still trying to put my finger on precisely why they are proving such an attraction. I would say that the only chance you have of getting around is to disengage brain and abandon your body to the elements. There is no other way you would get me jumping off a bridge into a freezing cold river in order to wade beneath plastic sheeting and scramble up the banks on the other side dragging half a tree trunk behind me. Nor, for that matter, would I have reacted so calmly in normal circumstances to other competitors whizzing past in their inflatable yellow kayaks yelling: "Did you know your's has a puncture, love?" Two hours later, with my throat feeling as rough as an electric sander, I was still removing green river sludge from my mouth.

But I have since entered others. Which just goes to prove that you don't have to be particularly fit or even a rugged outdoor type to do this adventure racing lark. Just barking mad.

Who to Contact: It helps to have some training in outdoor activities before you try some of the longer events, so call the Adventure Activities Authorities (01222 755715) for details of you local outdoor centre; for details of the Hi-Tec Adventure Series, call 01538 703203; the Ford Great Lakeland challenge involves canoeing across Lake Windermere, cycling over the steepest pass in the area and running up and down the highest peak (01889 582889); Salamon X-Adventure challenge involves abseiling, orienteering and the dubiously titled 'rope work,' such as swinging Tarzan-style across a 100 metre drop over a waterfall (0800 3894350).

GRASSBOARDING

The grassboard, or streetsurf as it is sometimes known, is both a surfboard that requires no ocean and a snowboard that requires no snow. It provides city dwellers with the means of testing their surf or snowboarding legs without having to trek further than the nearest park. Indeed, anyone who has tried snowboarding or surfing has a head start when it comes to learning this sport. The first ever grassboard was invented back in 1995 by Austrian snowboarders looking for a way to keep in shape once the snow disappeared. It was not long before surfers realised that they, too, could benefit. The boards have become increasingly high-tech since the early days. It is now a sport in its own right with regional and national leagues around the country. The most basic equipment, such as the board I use in my first lesson, has two wheels at the back and one at the front with footholds and a hand-held brake attached to the wheels. Still, it is daunting stuff free-wheeling down Primrose Hill in London on a busy lunchtime. I was told to bend my knees slightly and place the weight on my front leg, keeping my feet flat on the board. Lean right to turn left and left to turn right. The trick is to keep concentrating at all times. And watch out for stray pigeons.

Verdict: It is tough work dragging the board up and down the hill. Grassboarding will also help develop leg strength and co-ordination.

Who to Contact: For more information about grassboarding lessons and equipment, contact the London Beach Store, 178 Portobello Road, London, W11 (0207 243 2772).

HORSE RIDING

I discovered that I had been misinformed about horse riding during my youth. It is not, I discover years later, a bottom-spreading, thigh-thickening activity. Not that this was what prompted me to take lessons, you understand, but it was what had prevented me from carrying on with the sport as a teenager. Learning to ride, even as an adult, is relatively easy at schools approved by the British Horse Society where instructors, equipment and horses are regularly assessed to ensure they meet safety standards. With the help of a mounting block, I scramble up in ungainly fashion onto Betty, my horse for the day, and fidget apprehensively in the saddle until we're ready for the off. The most important thing for me to focus on, I am told, is my posture. "Imagine a plumb-line running from ear to shoulder and from hip to heel," said Wesley le Sondre of Ealing Riding School. "Open your hips, allow your lower legs to drop and push the weight down into your heels to stay balanced." Even the slightest shift in my position, such as leaning too far forward or gripping too hard with my knees, will unbalance the horse so remaining ramrod straight is paramount. Rhythm, it transpires, is the key to comfortable riding and as yet I don't have it. Perhaps the most profound benefit, at least for me, is the improved self-confidence that comes with knowing you are gradually exerting more control over something several times your size. And as a stress-buster it is second to none.

Judging by recent surveys plenty of other Britons think the same way. According to the British Equestrian Trade Association, the number of people who ride regularly increased by 400,000 to 2.4 million between 1996 and 1998. Interestingly, more than 70 per cent of those are women, although the proportion of male riders is beginning to rise steadily.

Verdict: As a means of getting fit, riding doesn't offer much aerobically (offering to muck out, apparently, is the best way to burn extra calories), but it will result in stronger buttock, thigh and trunk muscles without necessarily adding any bulk. The adductor muscles on the inside of the thighs work the hardest as you become more proficient because they are used to grip the horse but you will also rely on pelvic and back muscles as you control speed and direction.

Who to Contact: For more information on approved riding schools, contact the British Horse Society on 01926 707700. A full list of the 750 BHS schools can be found at www.bhs.org.uk

IN-LINE SKATING

Whatever you do, do not make the mistake of calling in-line skating 'roller-blading.' It is a registered trademark and you can only officially blade if you own an official pair of roller blades. All very confusing. As it turns out, if you once mastered good old-fashioned roller skating, as I did as a child, then you have a pretty good chance of being able to do either. Granted, I wasn't able to do the fancy forward and backward moves in my first lesson, but I could progress in a reasonably straight line which was way and above what I had hoped for. The idea, says our group instructor, is to keep your upper body relaxed and not to swing your arms vigorously across your body like a speed skater. Building speed is no problem, I found; stopping, however, is a little trickier. Protective gear is paramount at all levels but especially when you are a beginner and learning to do the scissor move is important as the criss-crossing of legs helps you to manoeuvre your limbs in the most constrained of areas.

Unfortunately many parks have now banned this sport because of the lack of control that happens when you reach top speed. This means that town dwellers are often pushed out onto the streets. If my beginner group is anything to go by, pedestrians beware.

Verdict: Half an hour of in-line skating can help you burn almost 400 calories as long as you keep going continually. It will also boost co-ordination, reflexes and, of course, balance.

Who to Contact: For a list of qualified instructors and more general information about in-line skating, write to British In-line skating Association, PO Box 145, Bicester, Oxon, OX6 4HH.

LAND YACHTING

A disused runway in Cambridge is hardly what I had in mind when I was invited to go yachting. But then I had never heard of yachting on land, a concept that is hard to grasp until you actually try it for yourself. The sport bears some similarities to both windsurfing and sailing and yet remains unique in that you stay firmly on land. Think of a windsurfer on wheels and you have an idea of what the vessel looks like. Naturally, it relies on blustery winds and the yacht won't budge an inch without them. At the top level, racing land yachts are made of fibreglass, costing up to £4,000 each and have the capacity to reach speeds of 95mph. Our beginners' versions, we were informed, would not exceed 45 mph. As I squeezed into the body of my boat and fixed my helmet, I began to wish the wind wasn't gusting quite as ferociously across the Cambridgeshire plains. I was told to hold onto a rope that connected to the sails so that I could adjust the length and to apply the right amount of pressure to the pedals beneath my feet to manoeuvre the vessel. Oh yes, it sounds simple. But one push from my instructor and I was sailing half way back to London, squealing pathetically as I lost any control I thought I'd had. In common with most beginners, I committed the cardinal sin of tugging harder on the rope the more I panicked which meant I moved with even greater haste. Finally, I rolled to a halt having unexpectedly turned into the wind. Keeping us within the confines of a smaller area seemed a safer idea and next we were to wind our way around a figure-of-eight course marked with cones.

By the end of the afternoon we were racing around them, taking corners on two wheels such was our progress. A second one-day course and we would qualify for the level-one landyachting certificate; complete a further two levels and you could apply for a pilot's racing licence. Joining a club is the best and most economical way to learn since you will be covered for insurance as well as instruction.

Verdict: Tough on the upper body. Age and fitness are no barrier. One member of the British team is 74-years-old.

Who to Contact: For information about various clubs, send an SAE to the British Federation of Sand and Land Yacht Clubs, 23 Piper Drive, Long Whatton, Loughborough, LE12 5DJ; for information about Windsport introductory days, call 01480 812288.

PARK CIRCUITS

One of the hottest classes in London last year was a military-style workout held in the capital's parks where, at the crack of dawn, former army PT instructors put gluttons for punishment through their paces. Its greatest appeal isn't that it is markedly different in content from any other circuit, but that it is staged outdoors, a novelty for the closeted gym generation.

In London, daily circuit sessions take place at various venues including Hyde Park where I signed up for an hour-long Saturday morning workout and other parks and commons. Bristol, Leeds and Manchester are the latest venues to be added and training British Military Fitness-style will truly spread nationwide throughout 2000.

There are regular week-long trekking trips to Wales and Nepal, too, where you can spend your holiday being bullied into shape. The idea for an outdoor military exercise programme based on the type of training given to army cadets was that of Robin Cope, himself an ex-Army fitness instructor, who was responsible for putting Tom Hanks and the cast through their paces in preparation for the film 'Saving Private Ryan.'

The circuit covers around three miles, although the format differs daily so regulars never know precisely what to expect. All recruits are handed a bib and initially directed to a coned-off area to warm up. This, it turned out, was the easy part. Run round, touching our toes or lifting our knees up to our chests responding to commands from Cope and his two ex-military assistants. Even in the warm-up slouchers are ordered to do a 50 metre sprint while the rest of the group hovers mid-sit-up, waiting for their return. And when the circuit got started for real, things got harder. Every few minutes we stopped to perform another set of conditioning exercises with the instructors bellowing mercilessly in our ears should we appear to be slacking.

Towards the end we were divided into two teams of ten for a 100 metre relay race over obstacles in which the batons were either half a tree trunk or a hefty leather medicine ball. Knock over one of the hurdles as you clambered under or over it and you were required to do 15 press-ups on the spot as your team-mates cursed and grumbled at you for slowing them down. A ten minute cool down and we were left, muscles a-quiver, to reflect on the morning's efforts. It was tough, but infinitely more enjoyable than being at the gym. Still, I was left with that odd sense of fulfilment you get after hammering yourself into the ground and promised to turn up again.

If the circuit has not yet made it to your neck of the woods, try creating your own. Sprinting between trees, stepping up onto park benches and doing star jumps on the park turf may attract bemused glances, but it breaks up the tedium of a run.

Verdict: Cope and his assistants showed no mercy, but the effects make it all worthwhile. The variety of upper and lower body exercises will keep your muscles from adapting to one movement and will make them work harder. As a result you will work harder than you would on, say, a run and the changes of pace will stop you getting bored. You will burn between 7.4 and 10.9 calories per minute.

Who to Contact: For more information, contact British Military Fitness on 0207 751 9742; email fitness@Britmilfit.com; www.britmilfit.com

ULTIMATE FRISBEE

The creators of Ultimate Frisbee, a group of students from Columbia High School, New Jersey, in the late 1960s, billed it as a friendly but competitive sport. Today the World Flying Disc Federation, the governing body of the mixed team game in which a ball is replaced by a Frisbee, upholds their original ideal. There is never a referee on pitch in this sport and its rule book states that fair play and gamesmanship between opposing sides should prevail in all games. "Competitive play is encouraged but never at the expense of respect between players, adherence to rules and basic joy of play," it states.

That aside, one of the sport's other big pulling points, says Ben Ravilious of the British Ultimate Federation, is that no beginner need feel intimidated when they turn up for the first time. "Anyone can play regardless of age, strength and experience," he says. "In fact technique is far more important than power when it comes to throwing a Frisbee." There are an estimated 100,000 people in 42 countries who currently play Ultimate and over 100 clubs are affiliated to the BUF in the UK. There is even a hotly contested world championship which attracted teams from 22 nations when it was held in Scotland in 1999. And Ultimate is also to be a demonstration medal sport at the 2001 World Games in Japan.

While in the early days, two teams of 30 played, gradually the rules evolved until it became the seven-a-side game played on a 70 by 40 yard section of a football pitch marked with end zones that it is today. Players aim to keep the Frisbee moving down field until a teammate catches it in the opponents' end zone and scores a point. Depending on the level of tournament, play continues until on team has scored 13 to 21 points in an international match which can take anything up to two hours.

Without an official to worry about, the game seems quirky the first time you watch or play. During a match, for example, any player holding the Frisbee has 10 seconds in which to pass it on to another team member. During that ten second time span, their defender from the opposition counts down loudly, partly in a bid to encourage a panicked pass, and if the Frisbee hasn't moved by the count of one, possession changes hands automatically.

In fitness terms, says Ravilious, it is tough, too, because you are sprinting up and down the pitch for much of the time. There are only loosely defined positions and players swap and change as is required throughout play, so must know how to defend and attack. Since flying discs can sometimes have a will of their own, self-defence from being hit on the back of the head with it as it drops with the wind is also important.

Verdict: According to Dr Paul Marfleet, medical advisor to the British Ultimate team, injuries from twisting and turning at speed are commonplace, but the grass burns incurred from diving for a catch are the most widespread. This game is tough but fun and far more demanding than throwing a Frisbee to your dog in the park.

Who to Contact: Write to The British Ultimate Federation at PO Box 1, Swan House, Leicester or email at buf@ultimateweb.co.uk; www.ultimateweb.co.uk; for details of a club in your area.

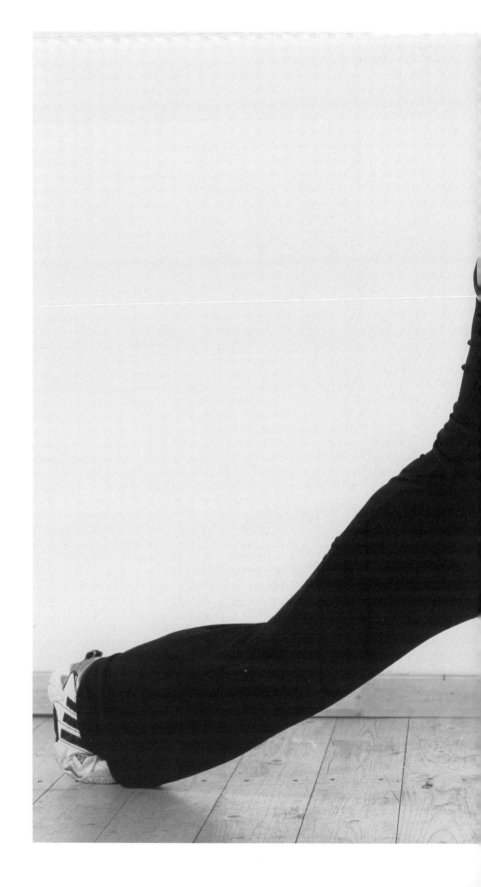

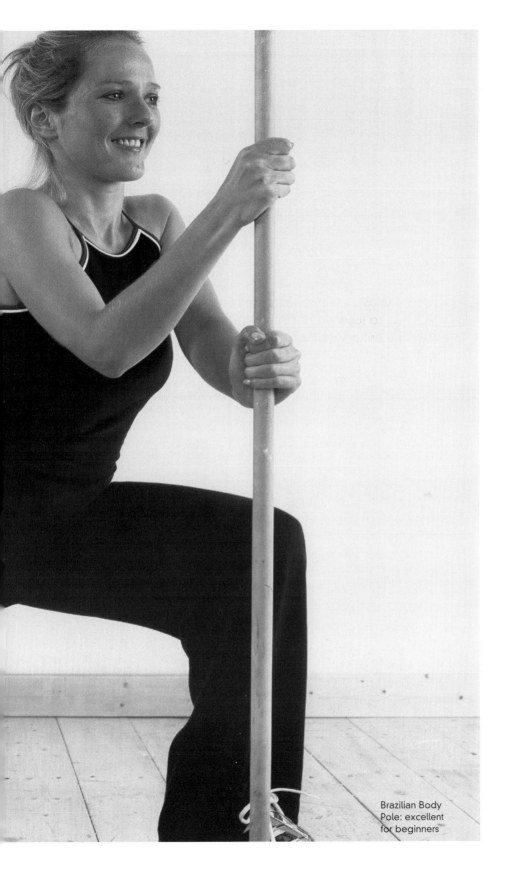

Brazilian Body
Pole: excellent
for beginners

STRENGTH AND FLEXIBILITY

Contrary to popular belief, strength training does not begin and end in the weights room. There is an increasingly diverse range of activities and classes designed to help you increase overall strength and improve muscle tone. And there is no doubt that it is a beneficial part of any exercise programme.

Most of the latest research shows that, for men and women, the quickest way to lose weight and tone up is to combine aerobic exercise, like swimming, running and cycling, with some resistance or weight training. While it is aerobic activities that are responsible for reducing excess body fat most quickly, it is strength work will improve muscle tone. the result is that the skin all over your body, but especially on the arms and legs will be pulled tighter across the firmer muscles, leaving you with a less flabby appearance. Train this way two to three times a week and you will soon see results.

A word about weight training for women who are sometimes put off the idea for fear or being transformed into the Incredible Hulk. In fact it remains one of the most effective ways to achieve a flattering shape. Rather than bulking up your body, making your upper arms and legs appear unfeminine, regular weight training will leave you looking more streamlined and toned. In men, it is the presence of high levels of the male hormone testosterone that results in them building bulk quickly with regular strength training. Women, however, are not naturally inclined to bulk up and a muscular appearance comes only with years of training with very heavy weights. The key is perform higher numbers of repetitions using lighter weights, called endurance weight training, not to lift the maximum weights you can manage which simply improves pure power.

Finally, a common mistake is to abandon stretching and flexibility exercises when embarking on a strength training programme. In fact, the two elements complement each other greatly which is why many of the new fitness classes like Pilates incorporate both strength and flexibility work in one session. Stretching helps to lengthen muscles and increase range of movement around a joint. In the long-term this will help to prevent the onset of degenerative diseases like arthritis in later life.

BODY PUMP

Body Pump classes are a relatively recent import from New Zealand, although the concept behind it is as old as the hills. This is a class in which weight training is done en masse in much the same way as it is done in a weights gym but with the addition of music and an instructor who tells you precisely what to do.

Equipment is a basic bar with discs of varying weights with a step stolen from Step Aerobics sessions and each move is choreographed to a funky beat. The idea, especially for newcomers, is to switch to lighter weights (for the upper body) and heavier weights (for the lower body) cramming aerobic exercise in between. Its incredible popularity no doubt stems from the recent research by scores of sports scientists that the most effective way to get rid of fat – and keep it off – is to combine resistance training with weights and aerobic workout. This class has both.

And the fact that it uses high repetitions rather means that you are unlikely to build bulk, only streamline and lengthen your muscles. Weight training has also been shown to improve bone density in legs, arms and backs of women who do it regularly according to the National Osteoporosis Society.

Most classes last an hour and cover every inch of muscle, including those you never thought you had. Unlike conventional aerobics you don't need to be fleet-footed to master Body Pump. The moves are uncomplicated so that even the most uncoordinated can keep up. Willpower, though, you will need in bundles.

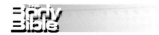

Verdict: One of the best all-round classes because it incorporates elements of aerobic and strength work.

Who to Contact: for more information about Body Pump classes call 0990 133434.

BRAZILIAN BODY POLE WORKOUT

Leading aerobics instructor Jayne Beck was jogging along a beach in Brazil when she spotted a crowd of locals working out with lumps of driftwood on the sand. This, she discovered, was working out Brazilian-style and when she returned to the UK, Beck selected the best of the moves she had seen and tried on holiday. The result was the Brazilian Body Pole Workout, a low-impact class that is suitable for all ages. Unsure about what to expect of a Body Pole session, I contacted Beck in advance to ask if there was anything I needed to bring. Although she provides special lightweight poles, moulded for easy handling,

I was told that a broom or mop handle would serve much the same purpose. During the warm-up Beck explained how it was important to focus on the various muscles I was using as I worked out as it would help to make the session more effective. After 15 minutes of conventional side-stepping to warm-up, we begin to use the pole in a series of intense stretches to ensure that our body alignment is spot on every time.

Such moves, says Beck, are ideal for elderly people who need to exercise to maintain mobility but who lack the confidence to move without something to support them. A lot of the exercises Beck demonstrates look familiar but when I come to try them with my pole I realise I have been doing them slightly wrong for years. In one movement we stretch the calf of each leg alternately by placing our hands on top of the pole in front of us and bending down slowly with a flexed knee, something I have done countless times before but which has never stretched my calf in quite the same way as this. We progress to muscular endurance exercises which involve a lot of bending, stepping and lifting.

The final high-energy phase is the abdominal section, which is mostly performed lying on a mat. Things seem much more sedate than my usual daily bout of fast and furious sit-ups, but I don't think I have ever worked my abdominal muscles as hard. By the time we come to the cool down, I am ready for it. Beck insists that, fitness aside, fun is the main aim of the Body Pole workout. It won't leave you sweating but you'll look at your Supermop in a new light.

Verdict: An excellent way for beginners to tone and stretch using the pole for balance.

Who to Contact: Jayne Beck's Brazilian Body Pole workout video is available from branches of WH Smith; call 01753 830176 for information about Body Pole master classes in your area.

DYNABAND WORKOUT

Along with retro adidas tracksuits, Dynabands are primitive pieces of exercise equipment that have somehow managed to make a comeback and re-assert their Seventies popularity in the new Millennium. Basically, the Dynaband is a giant rubber band that creates resistance and is used to build muscle strength in much the same way as weights.

The beauty of it is that it can be thrown into a handbag or suitcase so that you can take it with you when you travel and work out as you would at home. Freddie McGovern, a UK fitness instructor with the LA Fitness chain of gyms, uses Dynabands to help his clients get in shape before they go travelling either on business or for a holiday. and then makes sure they take the bands with them so that they don't return flabby and untoned. "I usually suggest people take one with them and try to exercise at least a few times while they are away. It is a shame to let all that hard work go to waste," he said.

Joining in one of McGovern's Dynaband workouts, we worked our way down the body in what transpired to be a tough, muscle trembling workout. To tone our buttocks, for example, we lay on our backs and fixed our bands around our feet. Then, with legs raised, we pushed outwards, working against the pull of the rubber for 12 repetitions. The tricep muscles in the back of the arm are worked by throwing one end of the band behind our backs and holding it firmly with the left hand, while pulling the right before swapping sides. A session lasts 50 minutes by which time we effectively worked on all the necessary body parts as well as marched and jogged on the spot to work up a sweat.

Verdict: For frequent travellers or even those who prefer to work out in the privacy of their own living room, resistance bands are a must.

Who to Contact: LA Fitness Clubs (0207 366 8080) run Dynaband classes; to purchase a Dynaband and workout booklet, call The Physical Company on 01628 520208.

FLEXABALL WORKOUT

Remember Spacehoppers, the orange balls with antennae handles on which you could sit and boing around the garden? Well, they're back and this time around adults are having all the fun. As a grown up version of its former self – same shape and, at 21 inches, a similar size – the born-again spacehopper is called a FlexaBall and is being introduced in exercise classes as a tool to firm up flabby parts.

Swiss physiotherapists first used inflatable balls with patients recovering from spinal injuries back in 1909 and Pilates experts sometimes include work with the FlexaBall as part of their posture treatment. Wendy Wright, a FlexaBall class instructor, admits that most people try it out of curiosity or fuelled with scepticism as to how an oversized beach ball can help propel them along to greater fitness. But they leave feeling they have worked their muscles harder than before and nearly everyone returns.

We began the workout with some gentle arm-circling to loosen up before using the ball for whole body stretches. Sitting on mats with our legs as far apart as possible, Wright instructed us to walk forwards with our fingertips until we could reach no further and then slowly rewind back to the starting position. As we progressed to the conditioning phase of the class, Wright explained why this is more than just a novelty piece of equipment.

The ball's very roundness and pliability mean the body has to work hard simply to stabilise itself and each balancing and strengthening exercise uses weak muscles that often remain untested in other workouts. Each movement in a body ball session is designed to strengthen these muscles so that they function more efficiently in everyday life, leading to better posture and fewer aches and pains. There is little chance of straining joints since the ball is positioned to support vulnerable areas in each move.

This makes it the perfect tool for elderly people with a fear of losing balance and also for pregnant women who usually have to give up abdominal exercise on hard surfaces at around month four of their pregnancy. In the USA, FlexaBall is used in ante-natal classes where many women find they can tone up comfortably until a few weeks before their baby is born. We tried push ups, thigh squeezes and countless other moves using the FlexaBall both as support and resistance. By the end of the strengthening phase of the class I was groaning with the effort of all the muscle clenching and squeezing we managed to fit into a 25-minute slot.

But our exertion was rewarded with a cool down in which draped ourselves over the ball. With my arms, legs and neck melting into the ball's surface I would have been quite happy never to have let go.

Verdict: An intense workout which is truly as effective at toning and strengthening muscles as any weights programme. And far more enjoyable.

Who to Contact: Call 0208 873 0966 for details of classes; To order a FlexaBall which comes with workout video and chart call 0207 704 2389 or 0208 878 6005.

HEALTHY BONES

The bone-thinning disease Osteoporosis will affect one in three women and one in 12 men at some time in their lives. Now comes the Healthy Bones class that aims to help fight off the disease with exercises specifically designed to combat brittle bones. Known as a silent epidemic because most people don't realise they have it until they suffer a fracture, Osteoporosis is caused by bone calcium being lost at a greater rate than it is replaced which results in bones becoming fragile and porous. UK rates of the disease are among the highest in Europe

Sports in which body weight is supported, such as swimming, do not have significant strengthening effects on bones. In 1998, researchers found that female swimmers and cyclists, for instance, had a similar bone mass to non-exercisers and another study in 1993 showed that the bone density of male cyclists who trained for ten hours every week was no better than that of sedentary men.

However, young women who did 50 jumps or skips a day for five months improved bone density in their hip by as much as ten percent according to one published paper while another reported that 30 minutes of jogging or weight training three times a week increased bone mass in the spine by an average two per cent.

Independent exercise scientists along with medical representatives from the charity the National Osteoporosis Society who helped research and prepare the programme say that each exercise incorporated into one of the hour-long classes is designed to strengthen bones in specific parts of the body.

Skipping, jumping jacks, resistance work in which you support your own body weight in exercises like the push up and weight training with body bars or mini dumb-bells, will all feature. The format of each class will change although specific elements will be retained. Members will also be given the option of having a bone scan to assess their current bone health as part of the package.

Verdict: Includes a fair amount of aerobic work as well as the strengthening exercise which adds variety. Suitable for all ages including the elderly and teenagers.

Who to Contact: For details of forthcoming Healthy Bone classes, call LA Fitness on 0207 366 8000 or Fitness First on 01202 390444; for a copy of the National Osteoporosis Society's booklets on exercise and bone health, send a cheque for £3.00 made payable to the NOS to PO Box 10, Radstock, Bath, BA3 3YB (01761 471771; E-mail: info@nos.org.uk)

PILATES

Pilates (pronounced pi-lah-tis) is a mind/body conditioning programme favoured by Hollywood stars. Its big attraction is that it works at lengthening and strengthening muscles so that you are left with a longer, leaner appearance with no added bulk. Many osteopaths and physiotherapists recommend Pilates as a good way to get rid of nagging back problems and poor posture and it is also very popular among dancers. It was originally devised in the 1920s by Joseph Pilates who, as a German prisoner of war in England, came up with the format to keep himself in trim. Now there are more than 500 studios in the USA and around 25 over here. Due to its sudden eruption on the fitness market in the UK, however, there are also plenty of rip-offs and many of the Pilates-style mat work classes are not as effective as the original version which relies on machines to get you working.

If you find a class via the Body Control Pilates Association, the recommended route, most sessions will start with gentle breathing and stretching exercises before moving on to equipment like the universal reformer, something which looks a like a mediaeval instrument of torture.

The exercises are surprisingly demanding and, since you are strapped into a device, there is little option for cheating. Consequently, those body parts that usually escape hard work find themselves put on the spot and you are warned that you may not find it easy to walk the morning after the first lesson.

Verdict: It is not a cheap way to get leaner – sessions cost around £25 a time with a qualified instructor – but if graceful lines and reduction of flab are what you are after then it is money well spent. Once you have learned the basics you can practice at home.

Who to Contact: The Body Control Pilates Association, 17 Queensberry Mews West, South Kensington, London, SW7 2DY (0870 169 0000) or www.bodycontrol.co.uk for details of classes; two videos – Body Control the Pilates Way and Pilates Weekly Workout (both £12.99 by Telstar) provide excellent tuition from leading UK experts Lynne Robinson and Gordon Thomson or try the books Body Control the Pilates Way by Lynne Robinson and Gordon Thomson (Boxtree Macmillan £9.99) or Pilates: The Way Forward by the same authors (Pan £12.99).

PSYCHOCALISTHENICS

Don't be put off by the name. This is a class that its orginators claim will help you get fit in 15 minutes a day. Thought you'd like that one.

Psychocalisthenics (or Pcals for short) is yoga with attitude, the thinking man's (or woman's) Pilates. It consists of a basic 23 postures derived from martial arts and yoga and combines breathing, stretching and relaxation techniques. Kate Stewart, my instructor, enthuses about the way it can help banish PMS, relieve headaches and worse, as well as improve co-ordination and balance.

But in 15 minutes? The difference, says Stewart, is in the way you are required to breathe in a Pcals session. Before we progress anywhere it is necessary that we master something called the integration breath which fully opens the lungs and must be repeated after every strenuous move. Then follow stretches for the entire human frame. We work the dorsal cavity (around the spine), the abdominal cavity, the back, legs, arms and finally the whole body. Most moves involve swooping our arms around in fast-moving extravagant gestures which undoubtedly helps to get rid of inhibition and tension. Next we repeat everything to music and then swoop into a cool down period.

Even after my first attempt at the workout I admit I was amazed at how fluidly I was able to move from one flowing position to the next. I felt invigorated and energised when I finished, not a feeling I always get after Step Aerobics. Be warned that the introductory class lasts five long hours in which you will swing and twirl yourself silly. But then it is recommended that you do the obligatory quarter of an hour a day to keep topped up. Can't be bad.

Verdict: You don't need co-ordination, strength or a great deal of flexibility to try this and yet all of those qualities will improve if you keep it up. Granted, it is a little peculiar. But for 15 minutes a day, the payback comes as a bargain.

Who to Contact: Send an SAE to MetaFitness, Squire's Hill House, Tilford, Surrey, GU10 2AD (01252 782661).

SAQ CONDITIONING

If you are wondering, SAQ stands for Speed, Agility and Quickness, the three qualities you will need if you want to improve at practically any sport.

While Joe Public exhausts himself with general aerobic and strength workouts he often neglects other important aspects of fitness, say the experts who devised this class, but the world's fittest and fastest are constantly looking for ways to enhance these three elements of their training. So, ssshhh, now you can get the edge over your squash partner too.

It was leading Nike-sponsored athletes like basketball star Michael Jordan, tennis player Mary Pierce, footballer Michael Owen and his teammates at Liverpool FC among others who contributed their training tips to form the basis of this class. Leading fitness trainers Ian Jackson and Morcombe Coulson then selected and adapted the best exercises used by elite sports stars and SAQ Conditioning was born.

Many of the moves teach you to do the things your body and mind won't forget even when they are exhausted. You will eventually become quicker just through habit, goes the theory. After a brief aerobic warm up we are told to find a partner and take up a position at one of several circuit stations around the room.

Two minutes at each activity and then a whistle will be blown to prompt us to move onto the next. My partner and I start with the Sidewinder, a piece of apparatus consisting of two velcro straps fixed to an elasticated cord that is strapped to each of our own ankles. The idea is to stand on one foot, stretching the other leg forward, back, up and down as your partner mirrors your actions. Sounds simple, but is hard work as your muscles are working against a resistance and you are also struggling to maintain balance. The Viper is next, a cruel exercise if ever there was one. It requires me to slip on a thick fabric belt with a long elastic lead at the back which is held by my partner to add resistance.

My task is to sprint towards one of four coloured cones as fast as I can when instructed. This takes speed, strength and a quick reaction time to execute well. Mini-hurdles, catching beanbags while jumping on a rubber cushion and visual acuity skills complete the circuit. It lasts one hour by which time you have worked most parts of your body and are thoroughly deserving of a relaxing stretch to cool down.

Verdict: Basically it trains the central nervous system which controls our subconscious reactions and allows us to respond quickly when a ball is thrown towards us, for example. However, even if competitive sport is not your thing, this is more fun than the average, run-of-the-mill circuit class.

Who to Contact: Call 01664 850951 for details of SAQ Conditioning classes in your area.

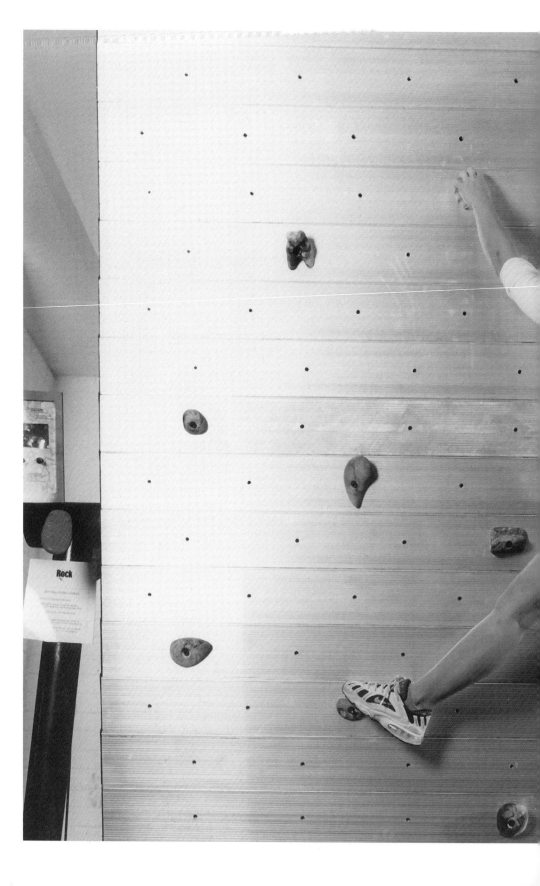

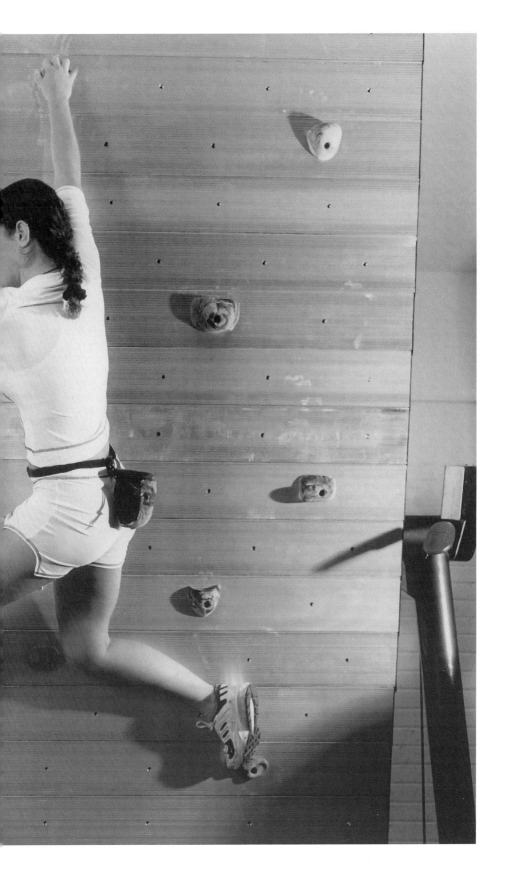

Indoor
Climbing:
plenty of
benefits

TRADITIONAL

In the pursuit of streamlined thighs and a satisfied soul, members of the gym generation are turning their backs on the treadmill and Stairmaster and reverting back to traditional activities like running, swimming and cycling to keep fit. UK Sport reports that more adults are now competing in these and other sports than they were ten years ago. And with the national curriculum also requiring more schools to add sport to their timetables after many briefly became competition-free zones in the 1980s, it can be expected that this trend will continue.

In terms of weight loss and toning, the benefits of taking part in a traditional activity are sometimes no greater than you would get if you completed a tough aerobics class in the same time. But since sport is unpredictable, your body will constantly be taken unawares, testing it's flexibility, strength, spatial awareness and reaction times to their limits. In addition, by switching the focus of your workout from the spirit-sapping battle to reduce the size of your derriere to a battle for self-improvement, be it a faster time or better score, the psychological benefits can be huge.

Research has proven, for instance, that people who play competitive sport at any level develop more positive mental and social qualities than those who do no exercise or work out solely at the gym. They become good at setting goals and working towards achieving them; they also develop discipline, organisational and social skills and are often better team players at work. A study by scientists at the Department of Applied Social Studies at Oxford University proved how participating in sport on a regular basis results in improved self-esteem in girls.

The sheer number and variety of sports clubs in the UK is vast and only a few are listed here. For information on all kinds of competitive sport, call UK Sport on 0207 380 8000.

BASKETBALL

This is one of the sports which has benefited greatly from National Lottery funding in recent years with around 10,000 outdoor basketball courts being put up in communities around the UK. Originally from the USA where it was first played in 1891, the game was invented by a Canadian doctor who wanted to develop a game that used gym apparatus and was played indoors.

To play at top level, height is an obvious advantage, but skill is more important quality if you are just interested in playing at a social level. Good hand-eye co-ordination, speedy reaction times and being fleet enough of foot to outwit your opponents are all vital to play well. Generally it is faster moving and more dynamic than netball with the rules dictating that there is less stopping and starting.

Getting started need not be expensive. You will need a decent pair of basketball or aerobic boots with ankle support and some cushioning and a pair of shorts. Hoops can be purchased from around £50 should you feel the urge to practice at home and even club fees are low with the cost to join in most training sessions being about £2.

If you get more serious about the sport and play for a team, you will be required to attend practice sessions once or twice a week and to play at weekends. The basketball season runs from September to April.

In spite of Michael Jordan's influence on the game which has enhanced its position in the men's sporting world, basketball has also the largest participation figures of any women's game in the world. It is well established as a women's sport in the UK and the women's English National Basketball League celebrates its 25th anniversary next year.

Verdict: Basketball is a technical game but also one which will test your endurance capacities to their limits – you spend much of the duration of the game running up and down the court. Since the ball is relatively heavy, you will develop good upper body strength and power in the legs from jumping.

Who to Contact: The English Basketball Association (0113 236 1166) has details of the 800 plus senior clubs in the UK although you may also find that sports and leisure centres run their own friendly sides which are not affiliated to the EBA. Clubs often cater for mixed teams as well as single sex and encourage people to join as a group with friends.

BOXING/BOXERCISE

Jimmy Mac's Boxing Club in Camden, North London, is hardly the kind of place you would expect to find the beautiful and rich, yet it is there that Naomi Campbell and a host of other models from the Elite Model Management agency have been put through their paces by Mr Mac himself. Campbell enthuses about the benefits of boxing workouts in helping her keep her supermodel shape, saying "It's the best training ever. It makes me feel so fresh and I have never been so fit."

According to Mac, while the supermodels don't participate in competitive boxing training, they do work as hard as many boxers when they work out. Skipping, punching pads, torturous circuits and hundreds of press-ups and sit-ups are all essential elements of training. The gym relation, Boxercise, is usually held as a class and is run as a circuit with exercise stations of the various disciplines.

Although women have competed internationally for a long time, under Amateur Boxing Association (ABA) rules they were barred from sparring with other women in the ring until a few years ago. The rule changes have resulted in a sudden rise in interest in the women's game and many more women being attracted to Boxercise too.

It is important to wear loose-fitting, comfortable clothing which doesn't restrict movement and a pair of training shoes for the gym-based classes. If you choose to try the sport, the best place to start is an ABA club where group tuition costs from around £5 a session. Most clubs will supply protective equipment like headguards although you will need to invest in a mouthguard and, for women, chest protection. A skipping rope is a useful purchase as are training and sparring gloves.

Verdict: Regular boxing training results in high levels of aerobic fitness as well as all-over strength. In competitive boxing, only when you are fit enough will you be taught any technical moves. Over time, Boxercise can totally re-shape your body.

Who to Contact: British Boxing Board of Control (0207 403 5879); the Amateur Boxing Association (0208 778 0251); Women's International Boxing Federation (01465 632448); London Amateur Boxing Association for clubs in London (0207 252 7008).

CROQUET

Keen to shed its image as a game played only by the well-heeled on manicured lawns in genteel surroundings, the Croquet Association is billing the game as one that can be played by the hoi poloi too. The message is getting across. Over 400,000 people from all walks of life are playing regularly and a lot of young players are being introduced to the game at schools. Lessons are also being held at sports centres and gyms around the UK.

Richard Brand, the instructor on my six-week beginners' course, explains that two forms of the game are played regularly in this country. Association Croquet, the more difficult to learn, is played to international level while a simpler version, Golf Croquet, is much easier to pick up. The bad news is you must learn the longer game before trying the shorter.

Hitting the ball with the flattened end of the mallet is surprisingly easy once you have mastered the golden rule of not lifting your head when you take a shot which causes you to apply top-spin to the ball and send it hurtling off track. Grasping the rules, however, is more difficult. The object of the game is to outwit your opponent by manoeuvring two differently coloured balls, black and blue versus red and yellow, through a series of six hoops. Trying to keep your ball in play for as long as possible, either by hitting it through a hoop (which gains you a point and one extra stroke) or by performing what is known as a 'roquet' shot in which your ball hits another ball and earns you two free strokes, you must follow a set course, going through each of the hoops twice, both on the way round and on the way back, and ending up at a centre peg.

Croquet it is known to date back to the 14th century – it is believed that a French doctor devised the modern game in 1830 as a form of exercise for his patients. The All England Croquet and Lawn Tennis Association formalised its own rules in 1870 although at the end of the 19th century, tennis had become more popular in the UK. Today, equipment is not expensive – you can buy a whole set for four players for around £100.

Verdict: Croquet involves learning what, for most adults, are alien skills. In terms of calories burned and muscle fibres toned, it is not of great help. But for stress relief and lots of laughter it is difficult to beat.

Who to Contact: For clubs and lessons, send an SAE to The Croquet Association, c/o The Hurlingham Club, Ranelagh Gardens London SW6 3PR (0207 736 3148).

CYCLING

Around 3.6 million people in the UK claim to cycle on a weekly basis. But with two million new bikes purchased each year that means a good few are rusting away in garden sheds. If your excuse is that you have nowhere to ride, there are currently 2,000 miles of cycle paths around Britain and with lottery funding the charity Sustrans is planning to increase that to 3,500 miles by the end of 2000. By 2005 there will be 8,000 miles of inter-linking off-road paths and 20 million of us will live within two miles of a designated cycle route. One of the main benefits of regular cycling is that it is a good way to get fit. Going to the gym is a means to an end but cycling serves the purpose of being a practical form of transport as well.

According to the Health Education Authority, cycling briskly for half an hour a day can halve the risk of heart disease. And while it is true that you never really forget how to ride a bike, if you find that your technique is a little lacklustre, then the British Cycling Federation runs Impruve groups around the UK where experts offer tips for beginners and those who want to sharpen up. In general, the rules are to aim for consistency on the pedals – don't pretend you are Chris Boardman on the downhill and then suffer the indignity of having to walk up a slope. "Aim for around 60 to 70 revolutions per minute because at that speed you will maximise blood flow to lower limbs and minimise tiredness," says Philip Ingram of the British Cycling Federation.

Make sure your seat position is correct. Your extended leg at the bottom of the pedal stroke should be almost straight. It will help to avoid leg cramps and increase pedalling efficiency. On a good bike that isn't too heavy and cumbersome, most of the effort comes from pedalling against wind resistance. The faster you pedal or the stronger the wind against you, the harder your muscles will work and the more calories you will burn. If you are thinking about buying a bike, make sure you visit a specialist bike shop where you will get advice about the height and type of frame you need. Opt for a bike with at least ten speeds so that you can adapt to changes in gradient and wind; if you plan to do a lot of off-road cycling you will need a bike with front and rear suspension. Expect to pay at least £200 for a bike with these features.

Verdict: Pedalling works most of the main muscles in the legs as well as the gluteus maximus (buttock) muscles in the push down phase. However, your heart, legs and lungs are the biggest beneficiaries if you cycle regularly. Coasting at three miles per hour will burn two calories a minute but if you keep going in the middle gear on variable terrain you will burn between seven and 15 calories per minute.

Who to Contact: Cyclists Touring Club on 01483 417217; for details of the British Cycling Federation's Impruve groups or to join a club, call 0161 230 2301; for maps and information about the Millennium cycle routes, call Sustrans on 01179 290888.

RECUMBENT CYCLING

If you have never seen one (and if you have you would remember), the recumbent bike is as its name suggests, a bike that has been rotated out of sorts. There are three wheels and the pedals are up where the front wheel should be. This type of bike has been around for years but only recently have they become the fitness tool of the trendy. In the USA, sales of recumbent bikes have doubled in the past two years and 40,000 were sold in 1999. One thing for sure, it is not the fact that they look cool that has people queuing up to ride them.

But at least they move quickly; even the most basic low-level bike can hit speeds of 55 miles per hour on flat ground and the world record for a human-powered land vehicle is set by a recumbent cyclist at almost 70 miles per hour. Needless to say, they are banned from regular cycle races. The rules are simple. You half-sit, half-lie in the cushioned seat so that your upper body relaxes. Most bikes are operated via hand-held brakes and to move faster you simply push your back further into the seat so that your legs have more range of movement. Manoeuvres can be tricky to grasp. Turning is cumbersome because of the wide-spread wheels.

The bike's low profile also means that you are virtually invisible to traffic. Many riders attach tall flags to the back of their seats to make sure they can be spotted. Personally, I preferred to stay out of public view altogether, tootling around the nearest park. Recumbents are suitable for all ages and are suitable for anyone who finds conventional cycling puts pressure on their back.

Verdict: The seated position means that your wrists, knees, shoulders and neck are under less strain than they are on a traditional bike. Research at the State University of New York recently showed that muscle usage is also different from conventional cycling. On these bikes your hamstrings and gluteus work harder than your hamstrings which makes it a better butt-firming exercise.

Who to Contact: London Recumbents on 0207 223 2533; the Cyclists Touring Club on 01483 417217.

FENCING

Cardio Fencing is a class that is popular in the States but, so far, has failed to make an impact over here. However, it did attract a flurry of interest last year when Catherine Zeta Jones wielded her sword opposite Antonio Banderas in the hit movie The Mask of Zorro. Now conventional fencing classes are also attracting newcomers, many of whom choose to join a club affiliated to the British Fencing Association.

While it is virtually impossible to learn this sport without intensive instruction from a qualified teacher, once you sign up for classes, progress can be swift. Some fencing clubs offer pay-as-you-go sessions for beginners in which you can have a lesson for as little as £5 - £7 with no obligation to continue if you decide it's not for you. In general, clubs will also loan or hire out fencing kit including jacket, trousers, foil and mask, which, if you did decide to invest in the full regalia, would set you back approximately £150. Learning privately is more costly with many coaches charging upwards of £40 per session.

Fencing can help to improve balance, poise, posture and cardiovascular fitness as well as toning underused muscles. It is particularly effective at strengthening abdominal muscles and those in the arm used to hold the foil. Upper back and leg muscles become stronger after repetitive lunging, although it is important to work at developing strength on the non-dominant fencing side (i.e: the side you don't thrust forward when thrusting the sword) otherwise you risk developing a lop-sided posture.

At top level, fencing is fast moving. So quick, in fact, that it requires the use of electronic monitoring equipment to assist judges in making their decisions. All movements in modern fencing are described in French and the terminology can be difficult to grasp at first but is easily picked up. Fencing is one of the few sports in which men and women can compete on an equal standing. What advantages men gain by their greater physical strength, women can usually match by being more fleet-footed and nifty across the ground.

Verdict: Fencing is often referred to as physical chess and after one session you will know why – it is as mentally challenging as it is physically and requires speedy reactions to dodge and avoid your opponent. Especially effective at working the back and abdominal muscles. You will definitely work up a sweat.

Who to Contact: British Fencing Association, 1 Baron's Gate, 33-35 Rothschild Road, London W4 5HT (0208 742 3032). Look out for fencing classes at gyms and health clubs too. Ragdale Hall Health Farm regularly holds fencing courses for its residents.

FOOTBALL

Confession time. Prior to last summer, my working knowledge of football amounted to what I had picked up on Saturday afternoons in my youth, occasionally accompanying my Dad to freeze on the terraces of The Hawthorns watching West Bromwich Albion play, and regular soccer reports from my Grandad, a statistician for Aston Villa, in the letters he sent to me when I was student.

I had kicked a ball before, of course, although, as far as I can remember, never in a straight line and had certainly never done anything remotely technical like trying to control a football with my head. But, oh, how I wished I had practised when it came to making my baptism to the game. Talk about being thrown in at the deep end. As one of a handful of novice female players, all journalists, invited for a kick around at the Bank of England sports ground in London which, incidentally, is where the England team train regularly, I had to make my debut under the watchful eye of, gulp, Kevin Keegan and several members of the Fulham Ladies squad.

As soon as we arrived, the England coach had us kitted out and running around the pitch, forwards, backwards and sideways, jumping and sprinting. And that was only the warm up. "Does David Beckham have to do this?" we panted as he lined us up to try some drills. Oh yes, and much more. To play football at any level, I learned, requires a degree of fitness way and above what is required to play most games at beginner's level. You must be flexible and fast with the endurance capacity of a long distance runner and yet must also keep on top of your technical skills so that you can out-perform the opposition.

While British men have been genetically programmed to be fully versed in the comings and goings of the Premiership and to know precisely what to do with a football for decades, for British women it is pretty much a whole new ball game. Women's football is huge in the USA and over two million girls in the UK now play soccer at school. In the UK, the sport is taking off and friendly, informal clubs as well as serious league competitions are springing up around the country. Some schools have also added football to girls' PE timetables. According to Kevin Keegan, an ardent supporter of the Fulham Ladies' side, the women's game is still in its infancy and is crying out for pro-active women to get their boots on and start up a side with friends. "The best idea, if you decide you like the game, is to set up a side with some friends and organise some local matches," he said.

He also stressed that, male or female, it can be fun and beneficial just to be left to your own devices and play ball with a friend to practice your skills. This is true, and by the end of my afternoon's coaching I was beginning to unearth the few Pele qualities that Keegan says lurk within us all. "On me 'ead, Kev, on me 'ead." Anywhere, in fact, but "on me chest." Ouch. How do those women do it?

Verdict: A 90 minute match is rather like a torturous circuit in which you are never sure how much recovery time you will have to catch your breath nor precisely what the next burst of activity will involve. For this reason you must be prepared for everything and train to improve skills, speed, mobility and endurance. At the top level, research has shown that an average midfield player covers around six miles running during one match – even the goalkeeper covers 4,000 metres. And players run at a cruising speed or at a sprint every 30 seconds.

Who to Contact: The Football Association on 0207 262 4542 for details of your local county football association and member clubs. Women should write to the Football Association (Women), 9 Willyotts Place, Potters Bar, Herts, EN6 2JD (01707 651840) for information about clubs.

INDOOR CLIMBING

At a London gym, two men were preparing to climb a mountain. Scafell Pike to be precise – all 3,208 feet of it. Neither was quite sure how long it would take them to reach the summit but they were quietly confident that they would make it. After all they conquered

Brent Knoll at 1,456 feet no problem a few weeks ago.

The Ten Peak challenge is an initiative by the climbing machine manufacturers Versaclimber to encourage more people to take up the sport. Entry to the national competition is free and there are no age limits – all you need is access to a Versaclimber machine in a gym, a little determination and a head for heights. The Versaclimber is like a high-tech step machine and was designed as a training tool for the NASA space programme ten years ago. The latest versions stand 96 inches high and precisely mimic the action of an elite climber.

Pedalling and pulling on the handles stimulates a pump system – oil is pumped from a reservoir or accumulator at the top of the machine – and the latest models allow you to increase or decrease resistance depending on how hard you want to work when climbing. In the Ten Peaks challenge you can enter your body weight before starting and the Versaclimber will inform you how many calories you have burned during the ascent. Competitors are also provided with detailed information about the distance they must cover from each peak which is entered into the machine . Once the summit is scaled, you record the time and enter it in a personal log which is kept at the gym before being entered in regional and national finals. The rules are simple – you must tackle ten of the UK's most famous hills and mountains during the competition which usually runs from March to September each year.

For the slightly less upwardly mobile, the Ten Towers Challenge runs at some gyms. Starting with Nelson's Column at 184 feet, you progress to the CN Tower in Toronto (1815 feet) via the Eiffel Tower (984 feet) and the Empire State Building (1040 feet) and six other towers.

Another indoor climbing challenge is The Rock, billed as the first virtual mountain to be installed in gyms and health clubs in the UK. This gleaming hulk of a machine is different from other indoor walls in that it is run by a computerised motor that is programmed to make the wall tilt, spin and rotate through 105 degrees and so re-create the demands of a real mountain. Designed in conjunction with the US national climbing team, the aluminium face of the Rock is 10ft 8in wide and 11ft 4in high – large enough for two people to climb at the same time. The surface rotates at different speeds while you climb and depending on your experience, you can position the hand and feet holds to make life easier.

The Rock's internal computer system contains details of some of the world's most famous climbs, from the north face of the Eiger to Base Camp Everest. If you choose one of these pre-set programmes, the Rock will automatically tilt and change pace to mimic every crag and overhang you would encounter on the real thing.

Verdict: While inner-city, indoor climbing may lack some of the appeal of a day spent on Snowdon itself, there are nevertheless plenty of benefits to be gained from reaching for new heights on a machine. Going up uses more calories than going forward so you will burn 420 calories in half an hour if you climb at 1.3 miles per hour. And because you feet never leave the pedals you avoid the pounding and jarring associated with some activities.

Who to Contact: For entry forms and information about the Ten Peaks or Ten Towers Challenges contact Versaclimber on 0121 561 2771; to find out where you can climb the Rock call 0208 994 3666; for details of other indoor climbing walls, send an SAE to the British Mountaineering Council, 177-179 Burton Road, Manchester, M20 2BB.

KORFBALL

Hmmm. A friendly sport this one. The moment I turned up for a training session with the Tooting Bec Korfball Club, I was informed about the sport's ability to improve your love life. The game, you see, is one of few in which men and women play together. And that is most definitely a big pull to the 20 to 30-year-olds who play it. To be honest I was a little bemused by the tales of who had been out with whom, who married whom and who else had slept with another team member. But once we got down to the business of playing the game itself, it was unexpectedly good fun. Korf incidentally is Dutch for basket and the game was first played in Holland at the beginning of the 20th century. The idea came about when a schoolteacher from Amsterdam wanted to add to his timetable a game that could be played by both boys and girls.

Today it is played in more than 40 countries. It has similarities to both netball and basketball, with the main visual difference being that goals are scored through the korf, a wicker basket suspended from a post. A pitch is divided into two sections with half a team, two men and two women, as attackers and the rest as defenders. Each attacking player is hounded by a defender from the opposition, who must be the same sex and preferably, a similar height, throughout the match. Unlike netball, anyone can shoot for a goal from within their half of the pitch and unlike basketball you cannot run or dribble with the ball. You also need to be somewhat adaptable with your skills since, after every two goals, players swap sides so that attackers move into defence and vice versa. It is exhausting work which demands you swerve and jump out of your opponent's way. Dodging the opposite sex is reserved purely for the hours of play, however. Post-match gossip revolves entirely around the Korfball couples.

Verdict: A game lasts 30 minutes each half, most of which is spent running around so it offers plenty of aerobic training. It will also boost hand-eye coordination, reaction times and speed if you play it regularly enough.

Who to Contact: Send an A4 SAE to The British Korfball Association, PO Box 179, Maidstone, Kent, ME14 1LU (01622 813115).

NETBALL

I hated netball at school not because it was a game played only by girls – at our school it wasn't – but because I found the rules intolerable. No running with the ball, no getting too close to your opponent and yet not getting too far away either. It was a game for those with inordinate amounts of patience combined with an ability to think on the spot so that you could outwit the opposition in an instant, neither of which I possessed in abundance. Years later I reluctantly tried it again, joining in a friendly match and discovered that those were predominantly the reasons I enjoyed playing the second time around.

I also found that, these days, women aren't the only ones playing the game – men, too, are joining in. Around 60,000 adults in the UK regularly play netball either as members of mixed or single sex teams and new leagues are being formed to cater for those taking it up for the first time since they left school. Rules remain the same whether there are men in the team or not and the only physical advantage males are likely to possess is that of being taller. Netball is largely a technical game which means that the quick-witted and nimble rather than the strong and powerful are at a greater advantage.

Since it was first played in Britain in 1895 after being invented in America a few years earlier, the basic rules have remained fairly constant. Most matches today are played on courts 100 foot by 50 foot, divided into thirds with a shooting semi-circle and post with hoop at each end. Teams of seven-a-side aim to score by placing the ball through their opponents' 15-inch diameter hoop. Each of the seven player's position has restricted access to certain parts of the court – the ball cannot be thrown across two thirds and only the goal shooter and goal attack can score a netball.

By necessity, play is fast and furious. A player can retain possession of the ball for only three seconds before having to pass it on to a team member in the same or adjacent section of the court. According to the All England Netball Association, the governing body of the sport in England, the pattern of play has developed in recent years so that it moves much more freely and smoothly than the stopping and starting game of old. And the game is even quicker when mixed teams are playing.

Netball is progressing in other ways too. In 1999, regulation pleated gym skirts and collared shirts were finally ditched and the England women's team's official kit is now a tight-fitting Lycra mini-dress with built-in knickers. Spectator figures, one presumes, are also set to soar.

Verdict: In a strenuous game you could burn around 500 calories and lose around one-and-a-half litres of fluid. Since it involves a lot of jumping, whatever your position, you will also work the quadricep, calf and hamstring muscles to propel yourself off the ground and land with ease.

Who to Contact: The All England Netball Association (01462 442344) has details of clubs for all levels.

POLO

Polo has undoubtedly suffered from its image as a sport for rich gents in silly trousers and riding boots. Think Prince Charles and James Hewitt.

However, more recently Polo matches have become the place to be seen for the young and beautiful. Think Liz Hurley, Hugh Grant and Caprice. Supermodel Jodie Kidd even played in the Women's World championship last year. Hence its soaring popularity among the hoi poloi and the reason why everyone suddenly wants to be seen to be doing, or at least spectating, it. Provided you can ride a horse (and you can still turn up for lessons even if you can't) the basic skills of the

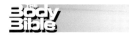

game are easy to pick up at lessons run by the Hurlingham Polo Association. Ten to 12 lessons at around £50 a shot will send you soaring into the heady realms of entry handicap minus-2 status. From there you can join a club.

A relatively new game to the UK is Arena Polo which is shorter and more user friendly than the traditional version. It is played on a smaller pitch with two teams of three players rather than four. To master the original you will need to swallow and digest the rule book. In a nutshell, a game is made up of seven minute chukkas (usually six of them). Play continues until a bell signals the end of each chukka when teams sit on the bench for three minutes (five at half time) and change ends if a goal has been scored. At elite level, to add to the melée, teams are handicapped and have goals awarded before they start. Confused you may be. But you will also be dazzled by the dashing figures gallivanting past you on horseback. Remember too that Susan Barrantes, the Duchess of York's late mother, once poised the rhetorical question "Doesn't everyone meet their husband at the Polo?" and, if you are single, I guarantee that you set off to try it at a gallop.

Verdict: Even at beginner's level you could be left as taut of thigh as a Jilly Cooper character. It is also an excellent way to build upper body strength and, since you are constantly reaching out at awkward angles, will improve flexibility.

Who to Contact: Send an SAE to the Hurlingham Polo Association, Winter Lake, Kirtlington, Oxford, OX5 3HG (01869 350044).

POWER WALKING

Scientists recently claimed that a daily stroll will not only help to keep off the flab, but can help prevent mental decay and loss of memory.

Researchers at the University of Illinois compared the effects of a walking programme over a toning and stretching regime on elderly volunteers. In the results of the study, published in Nature journal in 1999, they showed that the walkers performed far better in tests of mental agility than the stretching group. The reason, concluded the experts who headed the study, is that aerobic exercise like walking increases blood flow and oxygen supply to the brain which helps it to become more alert and efficient. As we get older, blood flow to the brain slowly decreases and brain cells shrink in size. But exercise can help halt this process. Indeed, walking was found to have a direct influence on the mental tasks controlled by the frontal and prefrontal cortex, the brain parts responsible for planning and memory among other vital functions.

For physical benefits and to protect health in the long-term, the further and more frequently you walk the better. In the Illinois study, participants started by walking for 15 minutes a day, three times a week and progressed gradually until they could manage a 45 to 60 minute jaunt three times a week. But if a 20 minute power walk at lunchtime or a ten minute stroll before a meeting is all you can manage, then you can still expect immediate psychological gains. Washington University researchers found that a brisk ten minute walk left subjects feeling more relaxed and energetic, while another study at Indiana University reviewed all the clinical evidence for and against walking and concluded that strolling at a reasonable pace for 20 minutes or longer was one of the easiest ways to boost mental health. In fact, they proved that the psychological benefits of regular exercise, including walking, produced effects comparable to the sort of improvements expected from a course of psychotherapy.

One of the most widely researched and publicised advantages of walking and other forms of aerobic activity is that it can raise blood levels of beta-endorphins, naturally occurring opiates that can heighten our mood. It is also known that other nerve chemicals like adrenaline, serotonin and dopamine are secreted in the brain during exercise, all of which have are required to produce a feeling of euphoria. And considering that a survey carried out by the British Heart Foundation recently revealed that full-time working women spend an average of 50 hours stuck behind their desks each week, a daily walk is bound to have positive effects. Getting your style right can prevent an unnecessary waste of energy and enable you to walk further without any more effort. "For a good walking posture, keep your back straight and imagine a line running from your ear through your shoulder, down to your hip and ankle," says Peter Wilmott, one of the 400 Walk Reebok instructors in the UK. "Keep your pelvis tucked in and your rib cage forward. Your body weight should fall slightly forward so that you can push off your toes."

If you are a novice walker, start at an easily manageable pace concentrating on taking deep breaths and perfecting your stance. As you get fitter, practice swinging your arms in time with your legs and increase your speed. Take shorter strides and remember to breathe rhythmically. If possible slip into a pair of sturdy walking shoes or trainers which provide support and cushioning if you plan to be out for 20 minutes or more and try to vary your terrain so that you are not stressing your joints repeatedly on hard surfaces like tarmac. No excuses. Take a hike.

Who to Contact: For details of Walk Reebok classes in your area, call 0113 237 1100.

RUGBY

Rugby, of course, used to be a game played only by men with oddly shaped balls. But while a schoolboy at Rugby School first picked up a ball and ran with it back in 1823 it has taken until fairly recently for women to do the same. In fact for the past five years rugby has been the fastest growing women's team sport with more than 10,000 women now playing on a regular basis in the 15-a-side Rugby Union game. The 13-a-side Rugby League – they split from Rugby Union when they decided to go professional – also caters for women.

Apart from the fact the the women's game in both codes remains largely self-funded, the rules and demands on the pitch are much the same. Across the board both codes suit a range of shapes and sizes since the different positions demand different physical strengths. It is not a sport to be taken lightly. Anyone can join a club, but once you commit yourself to regular training you will usually be required to turn up at least twice a week come rain or shine. Many who play claim it is as mentally challenging as anything else, which adds to its appeal.

Rugby has never been a sport devoid of injury risks which is why cauliflower ears are considered an integral part of the game. But it is not as dangerous as it is often portrayed. Nicola Phillips, chairperson of the Association of Chartered Physiotherapists in Sports Medicine and adviser to many leading rugby players, says that the last ten years have seen a marked change in the extent of injuries incurred by different team members. "In the past it was largely the backs who were at risk of getting injured, but now the forwards are much leaner and faster so they have more momentum across the field," she says. "This means there are more collisions and serious injuries throughout the team." 'Jersey finger' is the most common affliction. It occurs when a player grabs the jersey of a moving opponent and the tendons in his fingers pull away from the bones. Both Nike and adidas now market non-pull fabrics worn by international players which, they claim, should limit the extent of jersey finger injuries in the future.

Still, don't let the apparent brutality of it put you off. The game can be tremendously rewarding, both physically and socially. The cost of joining a club is relatively cheap compared with what you can fork out for gym membership – most charge an annual subscription fee along with a weekly charge for training which can be anything from £1 to £10. A decent pair of boots can be bought from around £40 and you will need protective gear, such as a mouthguard, if you begin to play regularly. But apart from that, a pair of shorts, t-shirt and track suit and you are all set for the scrum...

Verdict: The physical demands of rugby depend largely on the position you play. However, virtually everyone will develop speed, power and strength through running and tackling.

Who to Contact: Rugby Football Union (0208 892 2000) or Women's Rugby Football Union (01635 42333) for details of your nearest club. Beginners are always welcome and first sessions will consist of learning how to pass, tackle and handle the ball. For Rugby League it's best to contact BARLA (01484 544131) or the Rugby League headquarters (0113 232 9111).

RUNNING

There are two types of runner; those who like ploughing through mud, up hill and down dale. And those who don't. In the 1980s, the pavements and streets of this land were full of runners. We couldn't get enough of pounding along the roads and entering fun runs. At the end of the jogging boom, however, we were warned that slapping the ground with the soles of out feet was no good for our joints and inhaling traffic fumes about as beneficial to our lungs as a pack of Benson and Hedges.

By 1995, trail running, already an American obsession, was hailed as the healthiest way to run. In 2000, running anyhow and anywhere is fashionable. Trail running has a loyal band of followers and appeals to those who like the idea of escapism through sport as well as those with dodgy knees. But road running, albeit under the new banner of urban running, is making a comeback.

However you decide to do it, make sure you invest in a decent pair of trainers. (see Getting Started chapter p14). Run for an hour and your feet will pound the pavement up to 10,000 times. Each time your foot hits the ground, it absorbs three times your body weight and the shock reverberates through your legs and up to your spine.

Most running injuries are impact-related, a result of the added stress placed on the body when you grind out the miles. Well-cushioned shoes are a godsend to runners. Not only do they provide added comfort, but the latest technology means that advanced cushioning systems absorb a high percentage of the shock your body encounters when you run. Consult a specialist running shop for expert advice.

Trail Running

Hamsters might enjoy pitter-pattering aimlessly on a treadmill; human beings invariably don't. Only recently, however, has there been a backlash against the gym treadmill, that official route to tedium, and even film-stars like Meg Ryan are professing that the best way to get fit and conquer negativities within is to run outdoors, not on roads and pavements, but on park and woodland paths and trails. The benefits really are two-fold.

Not only do the hills, dips and flat stretches require you to change speed and use different muscles, but it really is easier to run for longer when the scenery is constantly changing. And if you don't trust your sense of adventure, a joint initiative between Runner's World magazine and adidas is marking out specific running trails around the country. Wherever you decide to do it, start by walking a route and build up to a jog over several weeks.

You will burn more calories running off-road than if you run on pavements or a treadmill because your legs have to work harder on soft ground. One study showed that runners covering one mile, even at a slow jog, on terrain like sand or mud used 148 calories, while those who ran the same distance on tarmac burned 123 calories. On average you will burn around 5.8 calories per hour for every pound of your body weight when you run or 3.1 if you walk. The basic running action also strengthens the iliopsoas muscles at the front of your hips and the gluteus maximus muscles in your bottom each time you take a step forward.

Who to Contact: Contact the Trail Running Association (0118 987 2736) or to join a running club call UK Athletics (0121 456 5098); for details of the adidas running trails call 0161 419 2500.

Urban Running

Trail running remains a suspect activity for the average city dweller. Why plough through mud and skip over tree roots with only a vague idea of where you are going when you can run directly from your own front door? The alternative for the streetwise and ballsy is urban running which, thankfully, is not half as bad for us as was once thought. According to Friends of the Earth (FoE), towns and cities do not even have the poorest air quality.

FoE spokesperson Roger Hickman says that by far the most damaging if you are exercising outside is a high ozone level which is usually found in rural areas. Dartmoor, the Suffolk Coast, the South Downs and parts of the Peak District National Park regularly record the highest ozone levels in the UK.

Even tarmac and pavements offer no greater injury risks to our joints than bumpy, uneven trails. "The extent of impact injuries from road running is about the same as those that result from twisting and turning injuries off-road. Make sure you wear a well-constructed, cushioned pair of shoes if you run on the roads a lot," says Trevor Prior, podiatrist to leading athletes.

"It helps to vary terrain if you can, but most people get injured because they don't replace their running shoes often enough, not because of an unforgiving surface. Shoes should be replaced every 300 to 500 miles for maximum protection." General safety rules include never wearing headphones, always donning reflective gear in the dark and trying to do several shorter routes from your house rather than one long run. Aaah. Concrete and traffic fumes. Don'tcha just love 'em?

Who to Contact: London-based runners can join a group which will meet at 6.30pm every Tuesday at NikeTown, Oxford Circus (0207 612 0800) for city centre runs; to join a road running club, call UK Athletics on 0121 456 5098.

SWIMMING

Nearly ten million Britons take to the water regularly, making it the nation's favourite sporting pastime. Swimming has undergone something of a revolution in the last 20 years and the techniques you may have mastered for the school gala have been overhauled and finely tweaked into a new range of strokes designed to get you through the water as quickly as possible with the minimum of effort.

According to leading swim coaches, most people who swim regularly don't get the most out of their time in the pool because they can't manage to keep swimming continuously for more than 20 minutes at a time. The reason for this is bad habits picked up over the years which hamper technique.

Making a significant change to your stroke is difficult without the help of someone at pool side to analyse your style and diagnose particular problems. But getting your stroke in order will immediately show results. Fewer jerky movements, less tension in the neck and shoulders and regular breathing improve speed as well as style. And just eight to ten lessons should be enough to get you into technically good shape.

For fitness results, Olympic coach David Lyles suggests a minimum of three 20 minute sessions in the pool a week. He also advises adding a progressive element by counting the number of strokes it takes you to complete a length and decreasing the number so that you get fitter without sacrificing your style.

Swimming is very good for the injury prone. Water acts as a giant cushion to save wear and tear on the body and, as you swim, the pressure of water can actually help to massage your muscles. Submerged in a swimming pool, you clock in at only one tenth of your normal weight which means there is very little impact on vulnerable joints. Medical experts often recommend swimming for people with arthritis or joint injuries.

For most people exercising in water is not solely related to the fact that it will help prevent sagging flesh and getting into great shape. The therapeutic benefits of water were recognised by the Romans and Greeks and for a holistic, overall mind/body workout, it is still considered the best place to start.

Alexander Technique

Remember that bad habits and poor technique will not only slow you down but can cause long-term health and posture problems. Steven Shaw has devised a revolutionary approach to swimming – The Shaw Method – based on the body awareness theories of the Alexander Technique. The most common problem with adults who learned to swim at school, says Shaw, is that they hold their heads up in the air which places tremendous pressure on the neck, shoulders and vertebrae which causes stiffness later on. There are many Shaw Technique instructors around the country who offer private or group lessons for complete beginners and people who can already swim.

"Your main aim should be to enjoy being in the water; to be confident enough to let yourself go and relax," says Shaw. "Don't try too hard but allow yourself to move more freely and your mind will follow. Once you are unrestricted you will swim like a dolphin." Well, after a few more lessons maybe...

Can't swim, won't swim?

Adult learn-to-swim classes are always popular, but choosing the right class can be an important factor in your future enjoyment of the sport. Go along and watch a class first of all to get an idea of what it involves. Make sure the teacher's instructions are clear and that the class isn't over-crowded with no more than ten learners in the water at a time. Beginners' lessons are usually held in a cordoned off area of a public pool towards the shallow end in thigh to waist-deep water and are generally run to suit everyone's pace of progress. You won't get left behind.

Lessons will include how to get safely in and out of the water and then how to practice gliding from the pool edge with floats. Only when you have mastered the arm and leg movements do you begin to learn the back stroke and front crawl techniques. Expect to have to sign up for a six to ten week course at a cost of £25 to £60. Classes usually last one hour with some including a free practice session afterwards.

Aquarobics

Don't despair – there are many water based options if you really don't like swimming or if it is taking longer than you expected to learn. Aquarobics, one of the most popular, was originally devised by sports physiotherapist Glenda Baum who developed a series of moves in water to aid athletes recovering from injury. Classes vary, but choose one that doesn't require you to get out of the pool mid-lesson (your muscles cool rapidly out of the water, leaving you more prone to injury). Most incorporate some form of resistance training using floats or other equipment which is great strength training work.

Verdict: A reasonably hard 20 minute swim will call on all the main muscles in the body to pull you through the water and some research has shown that because water provides 12 times the resistance of air, you can burn more calories and at a faster rate than if you were exercising back on terra firma. One study in New Jersey found that swimmers used 25 per cent more calories than they would if they had been running for the same amount of time.

Who to Contact: More than 2,000 swimming clubs are affiliated to the

Amateur Swimming Association (ASA) with many catering for every age group and taking part in regular galas. Call 01509 618700 for information. ASA coaches run stroke-improver or learn to swim courses at most pools, or, if you prefer individual attention, contact the leisure and amenities department of your local pool.

The Swimming Teachers Association (01922 645097) can also advise you about tuition near your home or for your nearest instructor in the Shaw Technique, call 0208 446 9442; Steven Shaw's book, The Art of Swimming (Ashgrove Publishing, £9.99) or video (Shaw Method Video, £14.95) are also available from the same number and at branches of Intersport around the UK.

TRAMPOLINING

"Do adults actually trampoline?" I asked hesitantly when I phoned the British Trampoline Federation enquiring about lessons. My concern when I ring to find out about lessons is that I will be turned down on account of my age.

But increasingly, I am told, people of more senior years do take to jumping about in the name of fitness. According to the federation's Jan Holmes, one fifth of the 50,000 Britons who trampoline regularly are over 20 and have taken up the sport for the first time. Since it is now part of the GCSE PE syllabus, many schools are also encouraging youngsters to try trampolining, so it looks set to bounce up the popularity stakes in the next few years.

I attended a session run by Ealing Borough Council in West London which, according to the instructors, regularly attracts upwards of 15 adults on weekdays. There are stringent safety rules to adhere to before you start.

Hair must be tied back, t-shirts tucked in, no jewellery is allowed (it might get caught in the webbing of the trampoline) and socks must be worn in case your toes get trapped and dislocated. Ouch. Spotters stand around the trampoline at all times to assist you should you bounce out of control and crash mats are positioned at each end for a soft, if misdirected, landing.

As you might expect from a sport that requires you to fly through the air at speed, accidents do happen although they are not quite as commonplace as one might imagine. There have been only 16 serious trampolining accidents since 1960 I am told as I clamber up. And with that I begin to bounce. Warm up by jumping up and down and aiming to hit the red cross at the centre of the bed each time, I am told. I could do this all day but the next command is to tuck jump, lifting my legs to my chest mid air and to half twist myself around after that. Next, I try a seat drop by flipping my legs in front of me and landing, if I am lucky, firmly on my bottom. Easy peasy.

The somersault, though, is a different kettle of fish and requires me to be manhandled by supporters through the entire move just so that I get the feeling of what it is like to gambol through the air. My confidence is bolstered afterwards when I am told that, with a few more sessions I will have reached my elementary badge status. A little more practice and I could put in for my GCSE qualification. Incentive indeed.

Verdict: You will puff but through concentration and mental effort, not aerobic debt. Beginners find it difficult to co-ordinate their bodies while bouncing and holding themselves in difficult positions at the same time, but it gets easier with practice. In time visual orientation, body strength and flexibility will also improve.

Who to Contact: The British Trampoline Federation, 146 Station Road, Harrow, Middlesex, HA1 1BH (0208 863 7278).

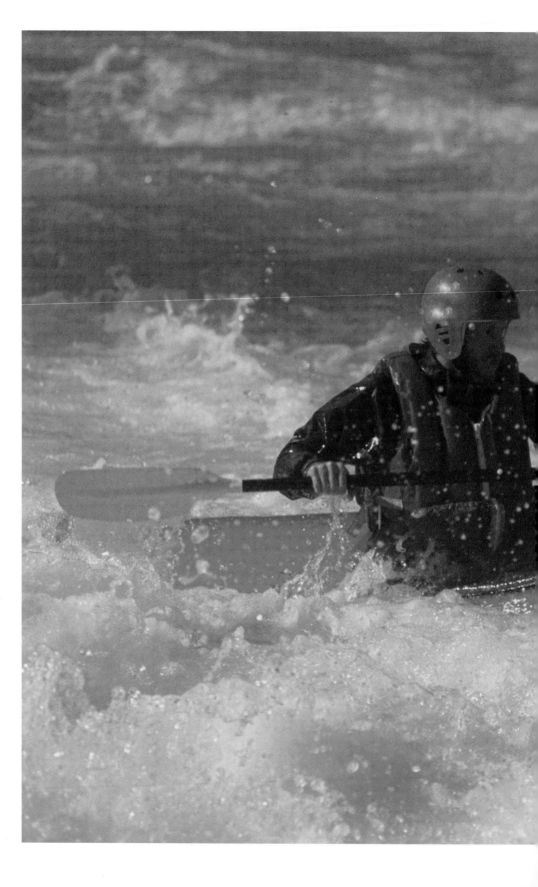

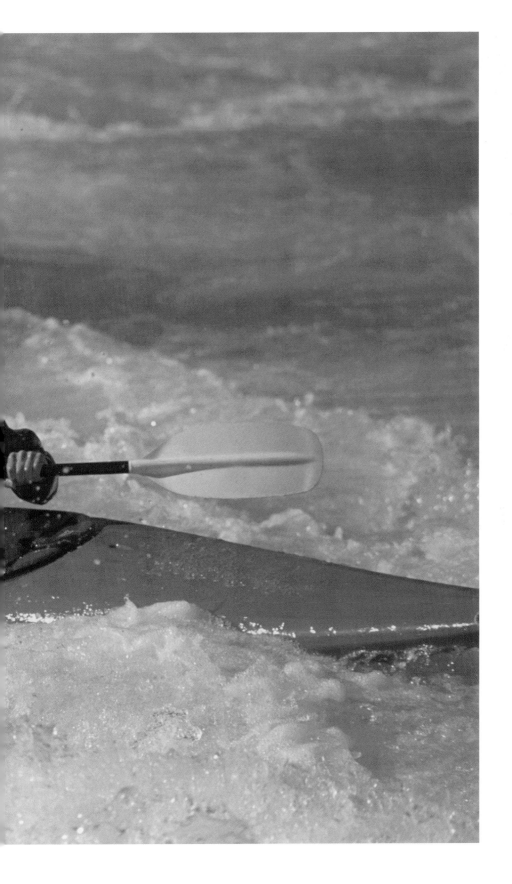

Canoeing:
has great
appeal

WATER FITNESS

Naturally, most water-based activities take place outdoors which, in the varying weather of these Isles, can be their biggest drawback. Unless the weather is good, there is little chance that you will get very far, especially as a beginner. Ferocious winds and driving rain are not the safest nor the most enjoyable conditions in which to take to the water for the first time. In some water sports, if the weather is too good and there is no wind to propel you from the shore, then you are pretty much spent too.

Still, weather aside, there are plenty of plus points to pursuing a water sport. The first is that, considering the value of equipment required to get going, most are reasonably cheap to try. Water sport centres generally hire out all the necessary equipment and any safety clothing and group lessons cut the cost of learning.

Always check that the watersports centre where you choose to learn (and there are plenty around the UK) provide instructors that are affiliated to an appropriate governing body or association. This will ensure that lessons are conducted to recognised safety standards and that you will be in no danger.

The centre itself should have some form of public liability insurance so that you will be covered if you are involved in an accident that could have been prevented by a more vigilant instructor. Check this when you ring up to book.

Water sports in the UK are definitely not for those who lack a sense of adventure, nor for that matter, are they suited to those with poor circulation who feel the cold. It can be perilous on the waves. So, for the less daring, I have included some indoor water activities which can be done in the confines of your local public pool.

AQUAGYM

All those who are paralysed with terror at the prospect of stripping to Lycra level in order to use the local weights room can now work at reducing their blubber in a far less conspicuous gym. The Aquagym is a unique British designed system that can be lowered into the deep end of a swimming pool and attached to the wall by giant suction pads. The beauty of the equipment which includes semi sub-aqua rowing, step climbing, abs unit, pulldown, strider and cycle, is undoubtedly the fact that only your head remains visible for the duration of a session. Many centres now stage Aquagym circuits such as the one in Leatherhead where I took the plunge.

Starting with a sedate jog into water wearing a specially designed aqua-belt which ensures you stay afloat and that your feet are hammering the ground as they do in regular jogging, you then proceed to one of the machines and begin an exhausting but gratifying circuit which lasts almost an hour. Unlike conventional multi-gym equipment, this has no weights, only plastic floats to push through the water. The water itself, provides three times the resistance of air so it is a natural form of strength training. Jogging between stations is obligatory so that you don't get cold. The body works deceptively hard in a class like this.

Because of the cooling effect of the water you don't sweat and the water also helps to massage your muscles so it is all too easy to push your body to its limits without realising it. Until you haul yourself out of the pool, that is, when your legs quiver.

Verdict: Far less daunting, although no less challenging, than the average gym circuit. An average one hour circuit in water would burn up to 600 calories provided you don't stop too often. Excellent for those who suffer joint pain as this is zero-impact.

Who to Contact: For Aquagym centres in your area call 01728 832755.

CANOEING

"Now let's try capsizing shall we?" says instructor Helen Barnes chirpily and only ten minutes after our beginners' group had first strapped ourselves into our vessels and ventured on to calm waters at the National Watersports Centre in Nottingham. Falling in is, of course, an inevitable part of the learning curve in most water sports but to do it voluntarily is a feat which requires considerably more strength of will than staying upright I learn.

One, two, three, a deep breath and there I was submerged beneath water and tugging at the various toggles that were fastening me in. It was as close to a near death experience as I have had and I eventually bobbed back to the surface cursing canoes, cold water and the day Helen Barnes was born.

Obviously some of our group fared even worse because they abandoned their shiny little plastic ships at that stage and wandered off for a warm shower. For the rest of us, with survival procedures taken care of, it was on with the lesson. On BCU approved courses you can learn the basics before progressing onto disciplines like slalom and sprint racing, rodeo canoeing which involves linking together a series of moves or just plain old river canoeing. The brave and unhinged in our group attempted the Olympic standard, man-made white water canoe course in the final half hour.

Barnes warned that there was a 99 per cent chance we would fall in and to beware of being dragged along with the current and flung against rocks. As we whooshed into the white froth she shouted out reassuringly that no one has yet died on a man-made course and that, anyway, there were plenty of people to rescue us. And so, at the mercy of the elements I felt somewhat secure. Admittedly I spent much of the journey going backwards, but I made it to the end without swallowing water. Would I do it again? Yup, but next time I'd make sure I kept my eyes open.

Verdict: In the UK, more than 500,000 people now canoe regularly, an increase of 25 per cent in four years, which speaks volumes for its appeal.

It is the stomach-knotting side of it that is undoubtedly the biggest attraction when it comes to tackling white water, but it will get you fit too. On average you will burn between 120 and 240 calories for every half an hour spent canoeing and, naturally, it strengthens your upper body.

Who to Contact: The British Canoe Union has details of clubs and facilities in your area – for an information pack send an SAE to: BCU John Duddesford House, Adbolton Lane, West Bridgford, Nottingham, NG2 5AS or email: info@bcu.org.uk; the BCU website is at www.bcu.org.uk. For details of lessons at the National Watersports Centre in Nottingham, call 0115 9821212.

SAILING

Sailing, once a pursuit of the wealthy, is now open to all and sundry who fancy a day on the ocean waves. Inspired by the announcement that 86,000 people are currently fully fledged members of the Royal Yachting Association, a figure that marks an increase in membership of 8,000 since 1996, and that many of them are spritely young things who don't live up to the Champagne Charlie image of old, I too signed up. There are more than 250 centres around the UK where you can enrol on a basic sailing course, although it is advisable to ensure the one you choose is approved by the RYA. Most introductory courses run as a weekend residential programme or over two weeks. The main disadvantage to sailing in the UK is, of course, the weather and while I picked a gloriously sunny day to hit the Solent, I can picture nothing more abysmal than having to spend a day on board a yacht when it is raining. One of the crew members teaching us the ropes spins the yarn of the time he fell overboard during an important competition and was bobbing in the Atlantic as his life passed before him in the form of his team mates sailing merrily on without him. Eventually, they realised he had toppled over, and returned to get him. But his tale put a whole new slant on the sport I had imagined would involve sipping a G&T once we had sheeted the sails. In fact, it is tough. All the pulling and manoeuvring and complicated orders will cause bruised knees and a weary demeanour. The upside was the odd snatches of stillness and quietness, save the lapping waves, which coincided with us taking a breather and encapsulated sailing's appeal in an instant. Rare moments indeed, but moments in which the rest of the human race, barring your crew mates, seems too far away to bother about.

Verdict: For a sociable activity, it is second to none since the boat won't sail without exemplary cooperation from everyone on board. The role you are assigned may seem alien as you set sail, but you soon learn that you are the final piece in a jigsaw, an essential key to enabling a huge hulking vessel move across the waves. And then your confidence soars. Physically more demanding than you might imagine too. Just don't forget your waterproofs and sunscreen.

Who to Contact: The Royal Yachting Association, RYA House, Romsey Road, Eastleigh, Hampshire, S050 9YA (01703 627400).

SURFING

Surfers are a hardy breed. In spite of the inclement weather on these isles, they reckon to lose no more than 14 days surfing in the five months of the UK season. And, of course, this hardiness translates as coolness in the world of watersports. Blond hunks and cool dudes go surfing, the car stickers should read. My instructor at the headquarters of the British Surfing Association on Fistral beach in Cornwall is tanned, blond and wears shades beneath the cloudy skies. He begins by giving us a run down on the various parts of the polystyrene boards we beginners will be using – there is the nose (at the front), the tail (back) and rails (sides) – and then we try standing on the boards on the sand. Boy this is easy.

First we learn to paddle, an essential part of the learning process as it enables us reach the necessary point to ride a wave. But by the time we reach the water, the waves seem a distant dream and the technique I had practiced on shore goes to pot. My timing, it seems, is the crux of my repeated failure to stand up on my board. First I choose the wrong wave, then the wrong second to catch it. Waves parted ever more ferociously overhead until everything clicked in an instant and I was upright. Balancing is another matter altogether and it took the best part of a day for me to be able to lay claim to the fact that I had headed in a straight line for more than ten metres. It is an unforgiving sport and one in which you must leave behind your inhibitions back in the beach hut where you get changed. Expect to be humiliated and exhausted. But all for a good reason.

Verdict: Cold, wet and infuriating. A sport which is undoubtedly more suited to temperate climes and one which makes you wonder why they ever introduced it over here in the first place. Yet once I had tried it I was hooked. Damn it.

Who to Contact: British Surfing Association, Champions Yard, Penzance, Cornwall, TR18 2TA (01736 360250).

UNDERWATER HOCKEY

There are times in which you seriously question whether your sanity has finally deserted you and my first game of under water hockey is one such occasion. Getting ready to play the game is a surreal experience in itself: pull protective hat tightly over your ears to prevent your eardrums bursting, wear socks in case fins start to rub, reinforced gloves in case knuckles get bashed and then smear spittle into your goggles to prevent them clouding over. Then without further ado, I insert snorkel in mouth and body in Acton Swimming Pool, West London where the London Ladies Octopush team train and jolly hockey sticks sub-aqua style. Since I doubt whether you have come across the intricate rules of this sport, let me enlighten you. This is a game played between two teams of six players who aim to flick or push a heavy lead puck into a three metre wide metal trough at the opposition's end of the pool. Sticks are replaced with 'pushers,' handmade wooden or plastic objects of no uniform shape or size but usually about one-foot long with an angled outside edge and a slightly curved handle. One side of the pusher is shaped like a meat cleaver, angled for easy flicking, and some players drill holes through the implement to lessen its resistance through water. It is currently played in 36 countries and Britain has a national league and knockout cup for male, female and junior sides. For me getting under water in the first place is an obstacle that takes several attempts to overcome.

With stomach skimming the pool floor I get a rude awakening to the true nature of Octopush. This game is brutal. Lungs burst as players fight bitterly to get possession of the puck and I admit I came up for air far more regularly than I needed to. I wanted to check that, if I needed to escape the melee beneath me, I could.

Verdict: Of course, having a large set of lungs helps as does being a reasonably strong swimmer. But do not be put off by the unusual nature of the game. It was the best time I had spent in a swimming pool in years. Not the best spectator sport...

Who to Contact: send an SAE to the Development Officer, British Octopush Association, Culver Farm, Old Compton Lane, Farnham, Surrey, GU9 8EJ.

WATER SKIING

The first shock to my system when I signed up to learn water-skiing is that invariably beginners are towed along not by a boat but by a series of wires.

Cheaper and more practical than hiring a boat, I am told, but I mean it is not quite the same is it? Still, zipped up in my rubber suit and awaiting instructions from the staff at a water sports centre off the M3 near London, I am filled with terror all the same. For some inexplicable reason this is one sport that has filled my nights with dread for a good week before I actually turn up to try it.

Being dragged along by any form of motorised pulley system symbolises a lack of control in my mind. I like to be sure that, if I fall flat on my face, it is as a result of my wrong doing, not that of a machine. But no getting out of it now and I attach the ungainly looking skis to the rubber on my feet and head for the water.

The idea is to crouch, knees to chest, while holding on to a metal bar attached to the side of the boat. Add speed and a fair degree of bobbing around on the surface and you have the ingredients of a splashing and sinking extravaganza.

Injuries, I am told are commonplace in this sport, and I should expect to come out not quite as intact as when I begin. At first, naivete plays a role and a false sense of security sends me on a wobbly but upright journey of some 20 metres or more. But then it is face plant after face plant and I am getting increasingly frustrated with boats, wires and rubber suits. My arms are limp, my spirit weak when suddenly towards the end of the afternoon I ski in calamitous style for a few minutes and the world is a wonderful place once again.

Verdict: There are almost 150 water skiing clubs in the UK where you can learn the ropes. Two lessons a week and within a month you should be fairly proficient, say the experts. However, dedication is a must as it can be an expensive hobby to pursue.

Who to Contact: British Water Ski Federation, 390 City Road, London, EC1V 2QA (0207 833 2855).

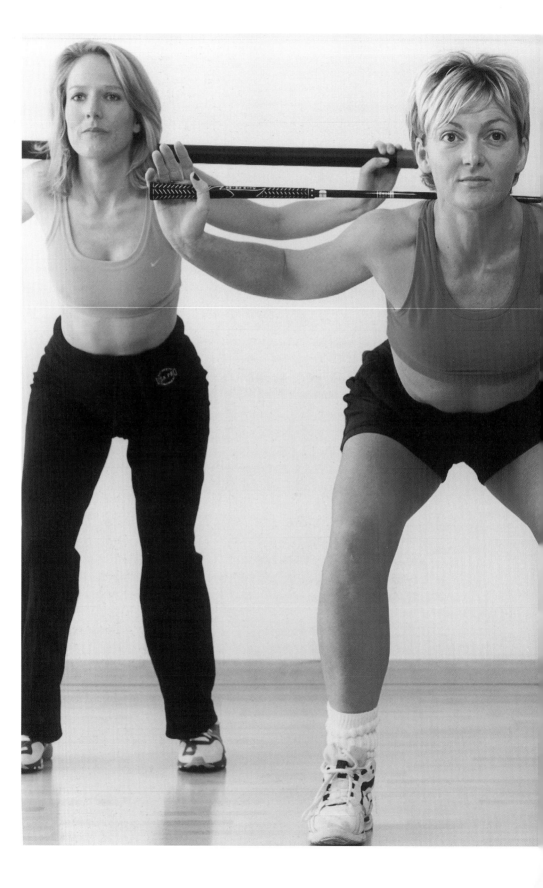

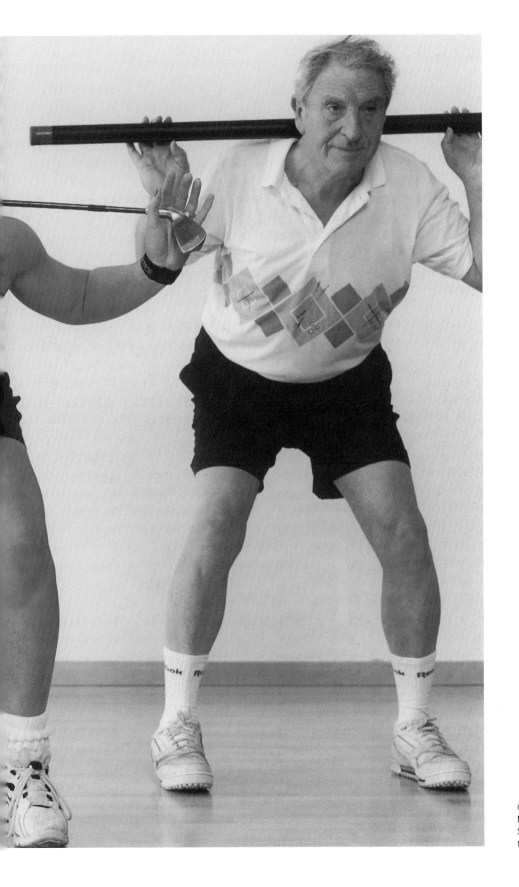

Golf-A-Cise:
Melissa
Scott leads
the way

WEIRD & WACKY

One of the most inspirational things about sourcing new fitness classes in the far reaches of the UK is that occasionally you come across one that defies convention to the hilt. So obscure are these forms of exercise that, on first hearing about them, you seriously question their validity and, sometimes, the sanity of the people who are promoting them.

Yet, dig a little deeper and you find that the physical merits of these workouts are as bona fide as any other and, at least for the people who take part regularly, provide as much enjoyment as more traditional means of staying in shape. They are never going to appeal to the masses, but these off-the-wall activities are there to be tried, if only once. Here are a few examples of the more unusual routes to slenderness currently on offer...

CATFLEXING

Catflexing is the latest fitness craze from across the pond where anyone after a Baywatch body is clamouring to get their hands on a copy of the book which advises ditching your dumbbells in favour of a feline friend. The idea was the brainchild of Californian-based fitness trainer, Stephanie Jackson, who started working out at home because she was bored with conventional gym sessions.

Picking up her moggy, Bad, one day she twigged that, at 8lbs, he made the perfect piece of weight training equipment. so she devised a 30 minute workout using exercises named the Cat Crunch and the Dead Cat Lift. After a few months of daily Catflexing Jackson was amazed at the changes both in her own physique and by the fact that her furry side-kick had also trimmed down.

"If your cat is out of shape, the muscle toning isometric exercises you perform in this programme could have benefits for him too," she enthuses. Jackson says the biggest advantage of working out like this is that it is free. All you need is motivation and a cat. "If you don't have a cat, see about borrowing your neighbour's," she says. "Even if you do have a cat, borrowing your neighbour's is not such a bad idea because your cat might not be in the mood to work out."

Such feline stubbornness is one reason why your Catflexing programme may flounder. Trying to persuade a reluctant Bagpuss to rise from his slumber, sit on your back and stay there while you perform three sets of 12 push ups is not easy.

Jackson offers helpful hints such as tempting kitty into the required position with a few strategically placed bite-sized pieces of his favourite snack. Having tried it with my cat, Eric, I discovered other drawbacks. The Seated Cat Raise involves sitting on the edge of a chair with your cat on your ankles slowly raising and lowering your legs. But I ended up with shredded thighs.

For the members of California's cat-loving population who have overcome these obstacles and persevered with the programme, there are now regular Catflexing competitions to find the most agile and muscular owner and kitty.

Jackson has also received letters from owners who have started flexing with other pets... anything from Yorkshire Terriers to lizards. But the workout is not without its opponents and Jackson has stirred up something of a cat fight with pet advocates who claim the whole idea is humiliating to animals. "Not so," says Jackson. "Do it properly and catflexing can be an uplifting experience for your cat."

Verdict: Those crazy Americans...

Who to Contact: Catflexing: A Cat Lover's Guide to Weightlifting, Aerobics and Stretching by Stephanie Jackson (Ten Speed Press, £12.99) is available by mail order on 001 800 841 2665.

GOLF-A-CISE

Poor golf. It might have Tiger Woods and a youthful new following at professional level but as for being good exercise, its image is still, ahem, something of a handicap: tubby businessmen, tight Pringle sweaters and putting the weight you may have walked off back on again at the 19th hole sounds more like the real story to me.

But golf is undergoing something of a make over thanks to instructor Melissa Scott who came up with the idea for Golf-A-Cise classes no less. Scott decided to construct a workout to help streamline golfers with a view to improving their game. It was she says, her own husband's poor golfing health habits – no warm-up or cool down and too many pints when he finished – that gave her the ammunition.

Through Golf-A-Cise she hopes to show that, while you don't have to be superfit to play a game it helps. After a gentle warm up of walking and stepping there follows a circuit comprising golf-related exercises, each designed to use the muscles that come into play when you swing or drive.

Golf clubs are used for specific exercises such as those to help develop rotation and range of movement in the spine. The circuit is repeated twice and Scott then takes the class through a series of stretching moves which she advises should be done before, during and after a round.

Since age is not a limiting factor, Golf-A-Cise is also helping introduce the joys of the fitness studio to a whole new public. Apart from their love of the game, the one thing her class members have in common is a previously held view that the inside of an aerobics studio was a no-go zone.

One regular in the class I tried at the Ealing Racquets and Healthtrack Club in London was 77. And loving every minute of the workout.

Scott says the ultimate aim is to ensure that for the three hours plus it takes them to complete a round, her golfers play to the best of their ability. And that, when they have a drink, they have deserved it.

Verdict: Look out for leg-warmers and leotards on the fairway.

Who to Contact: Melissa Scott trains several professional golfers. She can be contacted on 0208 421 2267.

HULA HOOP

My mum tells me I was destined to be a hula-hoop champion when, aged five or six, I would stand in the garden for hours twisting an enormous hoop around my waist. So, inspired by the prospect of unearthing this latent talent, I took a hula-hooping lesson. the first rule, I was told, was to purchase the right equipment. Just as Nike Air trainers are de rigeur for joggers, so the Wham-O Hoop is the in-thing for twirling.

Hoops have been around for years, but the Wham-O, complete with ball-bearings, is the very hula hoop that started the craze in the 1960s. Americans invented the craze after hearing how Australian children used a bamboo hoop during school PE lessons to keep fit. Within two years of being launched in the USA, the sales of the green and white striped Wham-O hoop had topped 100 million.

Experienced hoopers use it to tone their entire bodies, spiralling it around their ankles necks and arms or even trying the 'tush whirl' – an advanced exercise where you bend over from the waist so that your chest is parallel to the floor and rotate the hoop around your bottom. For me it was enough of a challenge to keep it at hip height for more than ten seconds at a time before it hurtled down to my feet. It was suggested I might be trying too hard and that I should put my hands on my head. It helped a little but more practice was needed.

Frustrations aside I imagine this would be a tremendously fun way to get fit. Grimly determined to perfect the art, I now wiggle as I walk for extra practice so that I will eventually attain tummy muscles of steel. In fact, keep it twirling continuously for ten to 15 minutes and you will burn 100 calories. Which is all very well, but I calculated that at my rate I was burning about four, Grrrr. Shoop, shoop, shoop....

Who to Contact: To purchase a Wham-O hula hoop, call 0161 633 9808.

KANGOO ROBICS

If the idea of in-line skating around your local park is enough to turn you scarlet just thinking about it, then read no further. Kangoo Robics is probably not for you. This emerging fitness craze which, admittedly, is taking a while to bounce off the ground since it first boinged into our vocabulary three years ago, is not one to try if you are a shrinking violet.

Kangoo Robic boots are basically skates with bounce; rather than roll yourself into shape, the idea is to spring along on the tough rubber structure fitted to their under-sole. The brainchild of Russian and Canadian runners who sold the idea to a Swiss businessman, they were originally designed to benefit injured athletes who required extra protection against hard surfaces when returning to training. Now fitness instructors around the UK are wearing the boots to put a spring in our step in aerobics classes as well as encouraging us to bounce around the local park in a pair.

When I borrowed a pair for an afternoon, I discovered, in fact, that much of the training benefit probably comes from the effort entailed in lifting yourself off the ground with the Kangoo Robic boots on your feet. Unlike skates, these things are of hefty construction, weighing around four kilograms per pair. The tread on the springy part avoids slipping and once you have got your balance and managed to stand up in them, moving forwards is surprisingly easy. The good thing is that, unlike travelling with wheels strapped to your feet, it is difficult to build up speed wearing these contraptions. Walking at a sedate pace first of all, I eventually plucked up courage to try a jog. The sensation was a little like trying to jog in a straight line on a bouncy castle when everyone else is jumping up and down beside you. Running style, too, must change.

Abdominal muscles must be tucked in and contracted as they form the body's centre of gravity and must be worked hard in order for you to maintain balance. Quite how hard I realised only the next day when my stomach felt as tender as it does when I have attempted a bout of sit-ups.

The boots are not foolproof and I found myself helter-skeltering onto a concrete path on more than one occasion during my debut run. I also attracted bemused stares from onlookers. One feels that a fitness studio may be the safest environment for the Kango craze. But pity the poor instructor who must control not only herself as she teeters mid-air on her bouncing boots, but the rest of the class trying to follow.

Verdict: According to researchers at Lausanne University Switzerland, the boots will help you to burn 50 per cent more calories than you would in an ordinary aerobics class held for the same amount of time. But you must first overcome feeling downright silly when you pull them on.

Who to Contact: To purchase a pair of Kangoo Robic boots and to find out more about classes and training call 01344 893173.

MIME

This is hardly your run of the mill fitness session. Yet an increasing number of stressed-out City executives are turning to mime classes to soothe both body and mind.

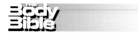

According to my instructor, John Mowat, at the City Literary Institute in London, many people are initially attracted to mime because they believe it will help them to relieve some of the emotions of a pent-up week. Like most newcomers, I had visions of being led through the two hours by a Marcel Marceau character dressed in striped top and black leggings who would show us how to blow up imaginary balloons and find our way out of a maze of make-believe walls.

But Mowat tells me that modern day mime is not necessarily silent and is far more varied than people imagine. To illustrate his point he breaks the ice by getting everyone to introduce themselves in their own gobbledygook language, using whole body movements to give their incomprehensible sentences added meaning. Then we are told to whiz around the room with sorrowful, crazy and lonely temperaments and finally to fall in love with the person standing next to us.

The trick is to avoid making eye contact until the end of each sketch when the whole class erupts into giggles. After two hours of running around and pretending to be someone else and trying on masks, I have to admit my energy levels were starting to flag. However, I also felt completely revitalised after what had been an unusually stressful week. Part of the appeal of the class was the lack of Lycra-clad bodies pounding themselves to exhaustion.

Before we leave, Mowat insists we give a verbal opinion of the class so that he can adapt future sessions if necessary. Half-an-hour later we are still hanging around, reliving the morning's experiences amid shrieks of laughter and chatter. Never get a mime class talking. You won't shut them up.

Verdict: It takes unforeseen courage to stand up in front of a room and rabbit away like a clanger. And even more nerve to fall in love with your classmate who was a stranger ten minutes ago. If you can do this, anything is possible.

Who to Contact: To find a mime class in your area call Total Theatre on 0207 729 7944 or the Midlands Arts Centre on 0121 440 3838; for details of the City Literary Institute's mime classes, call 0207 242 9872.

TALKING FRISBEE

Who would have thought that the humble yo-yo would have made a comeback in the late 1990s? But it did, thanks to the wizardry of manufacturers who came up with the format for an intelligent yo-yo. And according to marketing men, what high technology did for one spinning disc, it is set to do for another. Yup, we are about to enter the era of the Talking Frisbee.

At first glance it might look no more special than a smart version of the old favourite, but closer inspection reveals a single column of small red lights situated on the rounded lip and a lump underneath the centre of the disk.

And when you throw it the lights spell out a message which is programmed into a computer chip in the central lump which houses the batteries. The lights are sensitive to the frequency at which the Frisbee is spinning so that a message can quite clearly be read in daylight or darkness. At night the message leaves a trail like a shooting star. In daylight it sits closer to the edge of the frisbee.

The design is based on the same principle as the dot matrix system used on announcement boards, like those in the London Underground and other train stations. In this case, however, it is just a single layer of light-emitting diodes which is needed because the effect is achieved as it is spinning.

Its inventors explain that it takes advantage of the same time delay system between the eye and brain that allows us to watch films without noticing each individual frame. The chip can be programmed to synchronise the lights up to four rotations with eight or nine letters in each. The faster you throw the longer the word appears.

Be warned, however, that those who prefer to play catch in the park with a four-legged rather than a two legged friend should note that the durable moulded plastic from which the Talking disk is constructed may not be the kindest treat for your dog's gnashers. But worry not – for you there is the US-designed K-9 Frisbee to look out for. It is uniquely manufactured to soften as soon as it comes into contact with a dog's teeth. Oh, America.

Who to Contact: The Talking Frisbee costs from £20 and is available from The London Beach Store, 178 Portobello Road, London W11 0207 243 2772.

THE GYM ASTROLOGER

The UK's first in-gym astrologer, David Wells, is based at The Club at County Hall in London. Wells claims he can draw up your astrological birth chart, reveal the innermost secrets of your soul and then map out a health and fitness plan that will enhance both body and mind. Aah, you may well scoff. Precisely what I did before being unwittingly squeezed through the astrological mangle. As one who has always been cynical about what role, if any, the stars have to play in our destinies, I only ever resorted to a sort of comfort-reading of my horoscope when I felt down in the doldrums. I was doubtful that Wells could tell me much at all about my life when the only information I had provided was the date, time and place of my birth.

Breezing in for our 45 minute consultation, I expected a nice chat about where I had come from and where I was going. I was not prepared for the brutal unpeeling of my karmic layers which left me in tears.

This, I was told, is all part of the astrology package. In order to predict what sort of exercise would be most beneficial to me at this stage in my life, Wells said it was necessary to run through what had happened in my past. This he did with startling accuracy, reeling off my most significant emotional ups and downs, all but naming those involved, as if he was reading the pages from my diary. In rather mechanical fashion, on leaving I was handed an A4 print-out of my life's unfoldings entitled 'Know Thyself Peta Bee' and, among other things, was advised to switch from predominantly lung-busting forms of exercise to more spiritually soothing activities, like T'ai Chi, and to meditate daily.

Wells insists that one-on-one consultations are the only way to truly get to grips with your own life story. It is well worth the time but prepare yourself fully for the impact of it. I have followed his suggestions if only to give the next reincarnation of me an easier ride. Perhaps that is the whole idea.

Verdict: Emotionally draining.

Who to Contact: For more information call The Club at County Hall on 0207 928 4900 or to book a private assessment with David Wells, call 0777 5711956.

THE HORROR WORKOUT

Working out has just got scarier. So scary, in fact, that I had to be coaxed from behind a cushion to try the latest exercise sensation which wings its way to us from across the Atlantic. The Horror Workout is designed to unnerve you before you start exercising, to set your heart racing and your knees trembling even before you attempt to jog on the spot.

Based on an American idea, the theory is that you can frighten yourself into getting fit by watching ghoulish horror movies while you work out. Now a nationwide team of personal trainers, is introducing the concept to their clients in the UK.

London-based instructor Lisa Harman says that to get an effective workout and stay in the optimum fat-burning zone, your heart rate needs to maintain a level of 65 to 75 per cent of its maximum beats per minute.

Strapping on a heart rate monitor – which was used to determine how frantically my ticker was thumping – I sat down with a mug of caffeine and plonked myself in front of the TV to watch a 30 minute clip of The Exorcist. Before too long I was squealing and, after a few more cups of coffee, was sufficiently on edge to send my heart rate soaring. Harman dragged me off the sofa and on to the exercise cycle for a 45-minute workout

Part of the beauty of this regime, says Harman, is that people can scare themselves witless at home too. The idea is to choose a suitably scary film to get you in the mood – anything will do.

Whether the coffee was really necessary was debatable as I nipped back and forward to the bathroom, but I was assured that there are plenty of reasons why caffeine is beneficial when you are working out. Science, too, seems to suggest that it may help.

There is some, albeit inconclusive, evidence that drinking a few cups of coffee prior to physical activity can stimulate the body to use up fat more quickly according to sports scientists at the National Institute of Sports Medicine in London. The theory is that after drinking caffeine working muscles would utilise fat first and spare the body's glycogen stores for later use. Whatever the benefits, this is not good news for cowardy custards.

Verdict: Sports scientists claim that raising your heart rate before you work out may actually be self defeating, causing you to tire sooner so that you actually get less work done. Still, it is hair-raising good fun.

Who to Contact: For more information about the Horror Workout contact Active Fitness on 0208 968 0384; for details about Polar Heart Rate Monitors, call 01926 811611.

THE WACKY RACES

It is described as the ultimate test of endurance. a chance to prove once and for all whether you are man, woman or mouse. Organisers of the adidas Grizzly run held in Devon each year proudly publicise their event as 18 miles of vertical terrain and one mile of horizontal. The steepest part of the route, from a pebble beach, is labelled the stairway to heaven by past competitors. And yet the prize for the first runner home in this monster of marathons is a piece of driftwood. Second place gets a pebble.

As bizarre as it is physically testing, this is one of an increasing number of alternative fun-runs in the UK which are inspiring thousands of people to pull on their running shoes. But, while we Brits are gradually getting more experimental in our sporting endeavours, it seems we are lagging behind other nations when it comes to the most unusual race. In New Zealand, for example, there is an event called the Chunder run which requires you to run a mile, drink a pint and repeat four times.

Very few make it to the finish with the contents of their stomachs intact. New Zealand also holds the Undie 500 where competitors must wear only their underwear. While in the USA there is the Bare Buns race, an annual fun run held in a nudist camp. Clothing is optional, but most people choose to run in the buff, according to the organisers.

To find out about the adidas Grizzly Run call 0161 419 2500.

Meanwhile in the UK you can also try...

William Hill Man versus Horse. Held in Llanwrtyd Wells, Powys, in June. A £10,000 prize is on offer to anyone who can beat the first horse home in this 22-mile race held in Britain's smallest town. Alternatively, assemble a team of three who are fit enough to canter home before the horse and you could pocket £500.

Who to Contact: Gordon Green, Neuadd Arms Hotel, Llanwrtyd Wells, Powys, LD5 4RB

Race the Train. Held in Tywyn, Gwynedd in August. Recounting how you beat the Tywyn steam train over 14 miles 384 yards could impress your mates on a Saturday night. Most of this race is run on fields next to the rail track so that your competitor is always in view. According to the organisers, man has proven faster than locomotive on numerous occasions in the event's 15-year history. The course record (on two feet) is one hour and 19 minutes.

Who to Contact: Rotary Club of Tywyn, c/o 7 Yr Ynys, Faenol Isae, Tywyn, Gwynedd, LL3 0DW.

Meltham Maniac Mile. Held in Meltham, Yorkshire in July This event, run down a steep hill, boasts the 'fastest mile in the world record' at 3 minutes and 24 seconds. Even if leg speed is not your forte, you may find your pins can shift a bit when faced with a ten per cent decline. Race organisers suggest runners make arrangements for someone to greet them with a bucket of cold water at the finish.

"Entrants always need to cool their feet afterwards," they say. "The soles become red-hot because they are not used to slapping the tarmac at such a fast pace."

Who to Contact: Steve Renderson, 14 Ponyfield Close, Birkby, Huddersfield, Yorkshire, HD2 2BF.

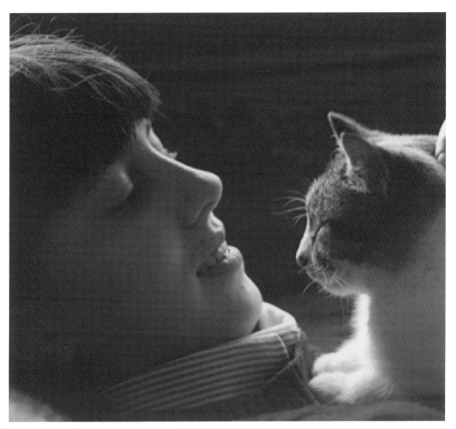

Getting the cat ready
for flexing!

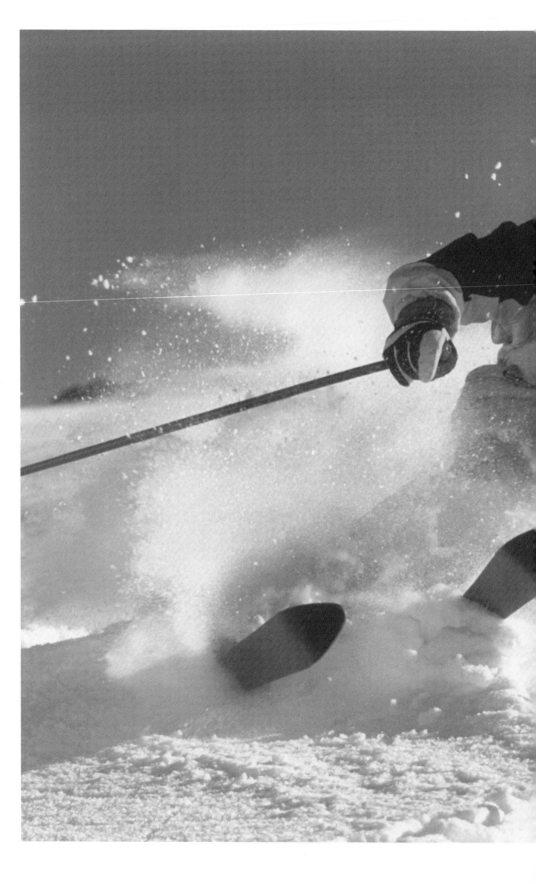

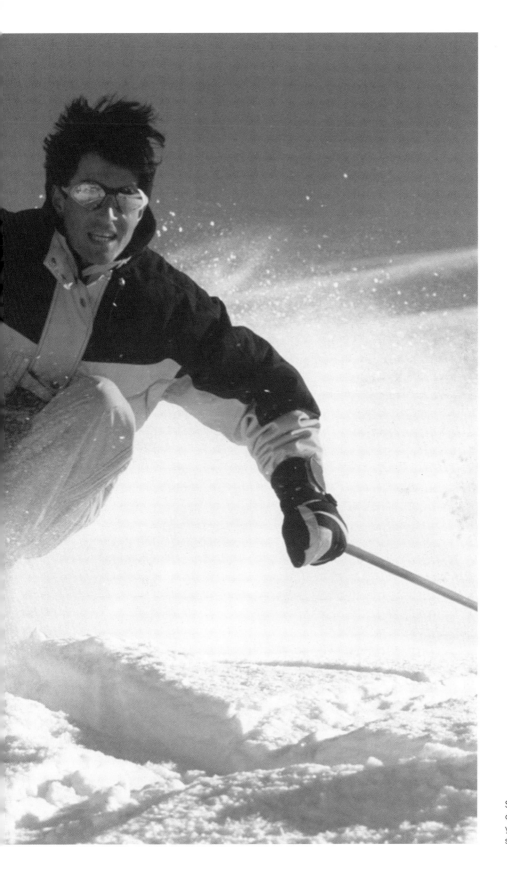

Skiing: worth a
dry run before
you hit the
slopes

WINTER SPORTS

For around 800,000 Britons, winter fitness annually involves packing a pair of salopettes and heading off to the slopes either in Europe or, increasingly, in North America. Most will return with limbs and joints as fully operational as before they went, but roughly one fifth will hobble back from an average five days spent on the snow with ailments ranging from sprains and fractures, with many more suffering from muscles knotted like pretzels.

The good news is that much of this post-piste agony can be avoided with a little forward planning. Skiing and snowboarding are both sports that require the body to move in ways that can hardly be considered natural and yet very few recreational skiers take the precaution of strengthening the muscles they will need to use before they go.

To lessen the risk of everything sliding downhill when you get there, Ski Fit classes held in many gyms are the perfect place to start in the months leading up to your holiday.

Another problem is altitude. It takes time to adjust to mountain mode and most people are not used to spending so much time starved of their usual oxygen intake. The result can be physical and mental exhaustion much sooner than expected – bumps, falls and bruises are almost inevitable.

Recent research has shown skiers that the third or fourth day of a week-long holiday on the slopes is the time you are most likely to incur an injury. Again, this is the effects of altitude taking its toll and experts advise sipping fluids regularly since dehydration is one of the main symptoms of altitude sickness.

Snow blindness is a painful condition which is often likened to having sand in the eyes and is caused by the cornea of the eye being forced to absorb too many UV rays. Skiing in sub-standard sunglasses or goggles which don't provide sufficient protection for your eyes is the usual cause. Even in mild cases it can result in headaches or muscular fatigue.

Finally, make sure you head outdoors with adequate sun protection. Not only does snow reflect up to 85 per cent of the sun's UV rays, but for every 1,000 metres you climb, the amount of UV radiation rises by up to 15 per cent.

This means that at an altitude of 3,000 metres, the sun is around 30 per cent more intense than it is at sea level. Over-exposure to sun is a common reason why skiers suffer on the slopes. Apply an SPF 15 glycerine and oil based sunscreen (water-based creams can freeze on the skin in sub-zero temperatures) to the most vulnerable areas like the face, eyelids, lips, ears and hands every two to three hours.

ICE SKATING

Lacing up my skates for my first ice skating lesson in 15 years, I mentally prepare myself for a cold, wet afternoon during which I could well lose my fingertips to a stray pair of blades. The good news, says Jason Blomfield a former British ice-dancing champion and my instructor, is that I can stand up. Most novice adult skaters have difficulty overcoming their fear of losing balance and of convincing themselves that they can stay upright for even a few seconds and spend the most part of their first lesson clinging to the barriers at the side of the rink. True, I am not yet re-enacting Torvill and Dean's Bolero, but at least I am vertical.

This sport has suffered in the popularity stakes in recent years, largely because its cousin, in-line skating, is hogging the limelight. Even so, I am one of 14 million Britons who give ice skating a go each year, many of them first-timers. The revival of interest, though slow, has resulted in some of the ice rinks that were closed down in the 1970s being re-opened by local authorities who see them as profitable ventures. The total number of public ice rinks in the UK now tops 70.

To encourage more people to take up the sport, the National Ice Skating Association launched Fun Skate two years ago, a nationally co-ordinated programme of lessons for beginners of all ages, backed with funding from UK Sport.

Private lessons are inexpensive, costing as little as £5 for 15 minutes. In mine, I am first taught how to skate in a straight line by bending one knee, pushing hard from my thigh and holding the other leg straight off the ground behind me

Skating is not an eyeballs out kind of sport – you may not even work up a sweat – but it is a good way to tighten the flabby bits on legs, buttocks and stomach. Just a simple turn requires contracting my tummy muscles in a controlled way, more akin to yoga.

Rather than burning calories, which it will do at a moderate rate of 50 in ten minutes, the biggest benefit for me was emotional relaxation, switching off from pressures of the outside world in a way that is never really possible at the gym. Circling the rink was truly therapeutic once I had rediscovered my sense of balance and I finished with the added satisfaction of knowing that I hadn't fallen flat on my face.

Verdict: Regular skating. two or three times a week, will eventually improve your stamina and endurance levels but improved flexibility and balance are the biggest advantages. Plus the fact that the rhythmic gliding movements are an excellent way to reduce stress

Who to Contact: For details of Fun Skate and other courses in your area, contact the National Ice Skating Association on 0207 613 1188; email: nisa@iceskating.demon.co.uk

SKIING

Thanks to the Snowdome, an indoor ski slope with real snow situated just off the M42, Tamworth in Staffordshire has become the epicentre of British skiing. Here, at Britain's first artificial snow centre, you will find 150 metres of puffy powder and absolute heaven for ski bums. A permanent covering of 16 centimetres of fresh snow, a ski lift to take you to the top of the mini-mountain and instructors to comment on your technique as you make your way down again, makes it a far more attractive option than the dingy old dry slopes that were previously the only option.

The temperature is chilly – although at four degrees centigrade and as cold as your fridge, it is probably not quite as arctic as Aviemore on a cold day – but provided you cover up in lots of layers, you won't notice the cold. This year two more Snowdome slopes are due to be opened, one in the South of England and one in the North.

At Tamworth, beginners can join in groups of one-to-one lessons run by England Ski Council qualified instructors where they are taught the basics of snow-ploughing, starting and stopping plus side-stepping up a slope to collect the ski/poles/glove you left behind when you fell. For me, the lesson was one in technique improvement since I have been skiing for years but, a bit like my driving, my skiing style has deteriorated due to bad habits. Nevertheless, I picked up some good tips from my instructor, particularly with regard to stretching and injury avoidance on the slopes

Admittedly, hobbling to the changing rooms with knotted muscles after an afternoon on Piste de Tamworth is not quite the same as heading back to the chalet in the Alps. But the Tyrol Bar is inviting all the same. Pash ze vin chaude.

Verdict: If you are planning a ski holiday or just want to hone up on your technique, it is worth at least one outing to an indoor snow

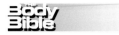

slope before you go. Dry slopes are popular but shorter – and you risk burning your legs when you fall over. Most people mistakenly regard skiing as a sport that strengthens only the legs, leaving one with tree-trunk thighs and bulging calf muscles.

In fact, it will improve strength, endurance, balance and flexibility all over. Strong stomach muscles are especially important both for preventing falls and for helping you to get back on your feet if you do tumble head over heels.

Also try Snowboarding

The young relation of skiing, it is hard to believe that snowboarding was only invented 30 years ago and even harder to believe that a sport now considered so hip was once called snurfing. A snurf was a board with no bindings, quite literally a surfboard on the snow (hence the name), but it has morphed into a sport that is the fastest growing winter activity in the UK.

Of the 80,000 people that head to the slopes each year, around 20 per cent now swap skis for boards each time. For die-hard skiers like myself the technique is alien and difficult to pick up. However, I am assured that I can learn the essential moves in a couple of lessons and that, in this regard, it is simpler than skiing for a beginner. First I must learn to skate on flat snow, then to side-step, turn and, whoa, I am away.

The jargon, though, is more difficult to grasp. Lost in lingo, I listen as one of Britain's leading young snowboarders, Victoria Jamieson, explains how I need to determine whether I am 'goofy' (ride with my right foot forward) or not and how I will eventually learn to ride 'Fakies' (backwards) and 'Big Air' (high jumps).

The thing to remember is that snowboarding is streetwise while skiing is still regarded by many as stylish; it is rough and tumble while skiing is graceful. And, alas, it is young while skiing is viewed as middle aged. Yup, according to statistics from the British Ski and Snowboard Federation, most people who take up snowboarding are no older than 34. It is worth a try, but bear in mind that your sell-by date will eventually be up.

Skiers on the other hand, carry on regardless of how well or badly the years treat them and wrinkles never look out of place. There is an enduring love/hate relationship between these two sports, so closely linked, yet miles apart in their appeal.

While you can try your hand at both, you must eventually decide where your heart truly lies. Ultimately, says Jamieson, you are one or the other

Who to Contact: The Tamworth Snowdome is at Leisure Island, River Drive, Tamworth, B79 7ND Group Lessons cost from £20 per person per hour

For booking details call 0990 000011; for details of lessons at dry slopes call the British Ski and Snowboard Federation on 01506 884343 (www.complete-skier.com) or the English Ski Council on 0121 501 2314.

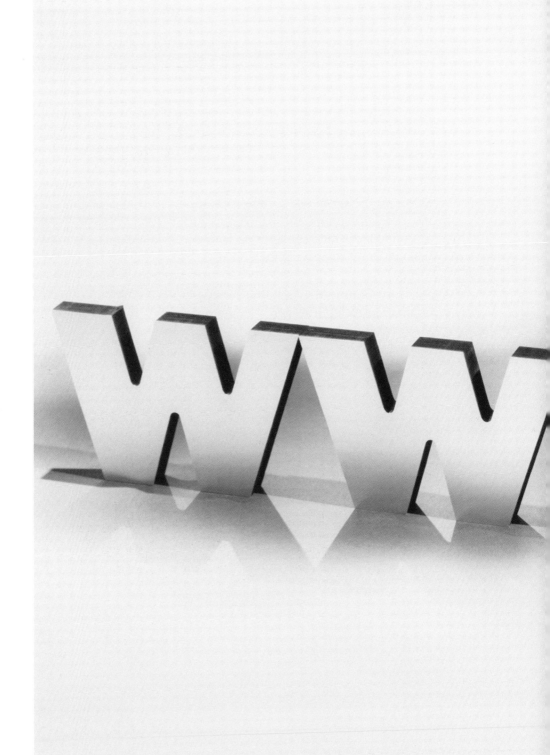

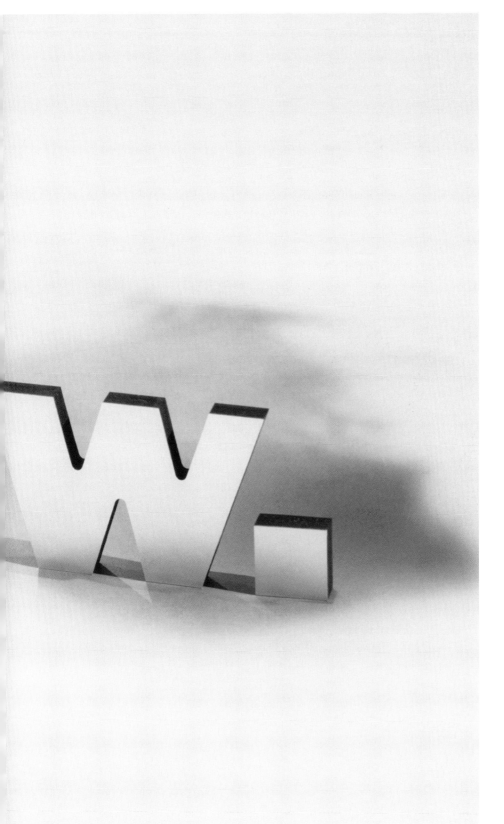

COMING SOON

You can even
use the web
to get fit these
days

COMING SOON

It would be fair to say that, when it comes to fitness classes, we British are suckers for anything that carries the star-spangled banner of approval. Virtually every class that makes an impact in gyms over here has already made one over there. Tae Bo, Spinning and Step Reebok, for example, were all tried and tested Stateside before making it big in the UK.

But in a business that is forever searching for more outlandish ways to make us flex our muscles, it makes sense for the fitness industry to keep an eye on what is happening in America. One doubts whether we will ever keep up with the relentless turn over of ideas that make brief appearances on US gym timetables each year, but doubtless there will be many that do survive the journey over the Atlantic. To tempt you, here are a few ways in which you could be working out.

ABS THIGHS AND GOSSIP

"Honey, I forgot my fishnets" sounds about as implausible an excuse for missing a workout as you can get. Especially if you are male. Not, however, at Crunch Gym in New York where stockings, high heels and shades replace Lycra and trainers as the compulsory get-up for the latest fitness sensation.

At Abs, Thighs and Gossip classes the emphasis is as much on glitz and glamour as on firming your derriere. Regulars slap on war paint like it's going out of style and take as much time getting dolled up as they might if they were attending a Hollywood premiere. The only person likely to upstage them is their instructor.

Wearing tight-fitting hot pants, a leopard skin headband and feather boa, Anthony Truly is the self-professed queen of the aerobics world and, as far as he knows, the only instructor who teaches wearing the uniform he dons for his day job – as a drag queen.

The exercises themselves are pretty unremarkable, with the usual steps, weights and mat format. But Truly puts his own spin on things and whoops his way through every track, swinging his ponytail around and checking on your technique. "Honey don't work too hard or your butt will look as good as mine," are typical of the comments he makes to regulars.

In the second half of the class, after 30 minutes of flexing biceps and performing squats and lunges by the dozen, Truly instructs everyone to stop, freshen up, take a breather and have a cup of tea. While everyone else slumps to the floor and performs light stretches as instructed, Truly uses the time to catch up on celebrity gossip and tittle tattle.

He even throws in some etiquette tips on how to behave at parties. "Don't bring uninvited guests to an office party and, although it's tempting, don't drink too much," he advises.

And, as if to prove that cross-dressing can really get you fit, Truly changes his outfit every week adding outrageous accessories to ensure his regulars don't find the class, ahem, a drag. A favourite is to perform press-ups wearing a pair of yellow rubber gloves. Marigold Aerobics? Could be the next fitness fad.

ON-LINE MR MOTIVATORS

If you harbour ambitions to attain a torso as exquisitely chiselled as a top athlete's then you will be pleased to learn that you can now call on leading fitness experts who will coax you into shape without ever having to step outside the door.

Personal trainers on the internet are the hottest fitness accessory and cost considerably less than the normal price of a real-life trainer but will give virtually the same service on the Web. The downside, obviously, is that with no one present to supervise you there is plenty of scope for playing Quake on the net instead of finishing your quota of situps.

So far, the best on-line training services are US-based but more and more UK trainers are offering their services. Most cost around £20 per month with special reductions for families and year memberships in some cases. Be warned that choosing a trainer from the net is not without its hazards – there is no agreed definition either here or in the States about who can call themselves a personal trainer, so always check for qualifications. Here is a guide to what's on offer:

www.fit-online.com Targeted at those who want to be more active without getting bored with their fitness programme. Certified US trainers evaluate your fitness and health status using a questionnaire before setting your programme.

www.fitsource.com Elizabeth Taylor is one of a lengthy list of celebrities to have employed this site's trainer, Xavier Carrica. Of all the on-line trainers he appears to be the most prolific and is very well-qualified. An impressive site in which a receptionist takes you on a tour of the club before Carrica questions you about fitness. He is a hard task master and keeps in touch by e-mail.

www.stonfitness.com Accredited physiologists prescribe tough sessions for your specific fitness weaknesses or aesthetic shortcomings. There is an optional three week introduction to exercise course from which you can progress to the likes of Great Legs or Butt Break workouts when you are ft enough. Six week customised courses are available to anyone wanting to improve in a particular sport like golf or tennis.

www.lifematters.com This offers free general advice about getting fit as well as subscriptions for working out with a trainer. There is also an open forum hosted by expert Jack Dixon to whom you can post your fitness queries. Things can get costly if you decide to take up a strength training programme combined with a nutrition consultation which will set you back around £60. This does include two e-mail follow-ups one of which, presumably, is to remind you that you are not yet sylph-like and should renew your subscription.

THE FOUR MINUTE WORKOUT

A fitness professor in America suggests that we can make ourselves fitter by doing only four minutes of exercise a day. Dr Robert Otto, of the Human Performance Laboratories, Adelphi University in New York, will doubtless become a millionaire if his calculations are correct, although, sadly, British experts are suspicious that his evidence is well-founded.

Otto's claim came after a study at the university, in which two groups of couch potatoes were asked to exercise to around 75 per cent of their maximum heart rate for six weeks. One group got to jog for 20 minutes on a treadmill while the other spent four minutes on a stationary bike with handlebars that move to work the upper body.

At the end of the study, the four-minute group had increased its oxygen consumption (VO2 Max), a measure of aerobic capacity by up to three per cent more than the luckless joggers. This, Otto suggested, could mean the end to self-imposed torture. However, British experts disagree. While the four minuters' aerobic capacity improved there was no improvement in their fat burning scores. Bob Smith, a sports physiologist at Loughborough University, says that "fat mobilisation is decreased compared with exercise that requires you to be on your feet for along time."

For gym regulars, stresses Otto, working out in four minute chunks is not a bad way to focus the mind. Psychologically, he claims, it is more beneficial than plugging in the Walkman and going through the motions in remote control for half an hour. And, of course, having a four minute deadline did wonders for Roger Bannister...

THE TWENTY FOUR HOUR GYM

Our nocturnal lifestyles are turning us into a nation of dimwits, experts warned in a study published in 1999. Miss one hour of the eight hours of sleep recommended by experts and you will drop one IQ point the following day; lose 15 points from an average 100-point IQ and you will be significantly closer to moron than MENSA.

But what does it do to your body? Hot on the heels of the Americans who with 24-hour everything must be galloping headlong towards imbecility, the UK has its first 24-hour gym.

The Club at County Hall in London is open all hours "to provide a convenient service for those who can't or don't choose to work out at regular hours." More are set to follow. Knackered you may be, but being tired is no longer an excuse for avoiding exercise.

However, what sounds like good news for your biceps could be bad news for your sanity. According to Dr Tom Mackay, a consultant in Sleep Medicine at Edinburgh Royal Infirmary. Getting on board the treadmill in the dead of the night will do you no good at all. It is, he says a fast route to social alienation and depletion of brain cells. "You are breaking your natural biorhythms," says Dr Mackay.

"You need time to recover mentally and physically from a day's work, so pumping iron or doing an aerobics class when subconsciously you want to be asleep can be counter-productive." There is a pre-programmed time for everything and, try doing it differently, your system goes haywire. The midnight workout, it seems, will take a few more years to be a hit on this side of the pond.

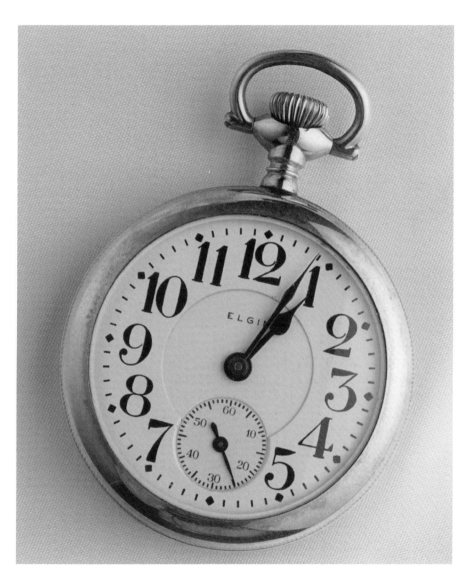

Take your pick
– four minutes
or 24 hours

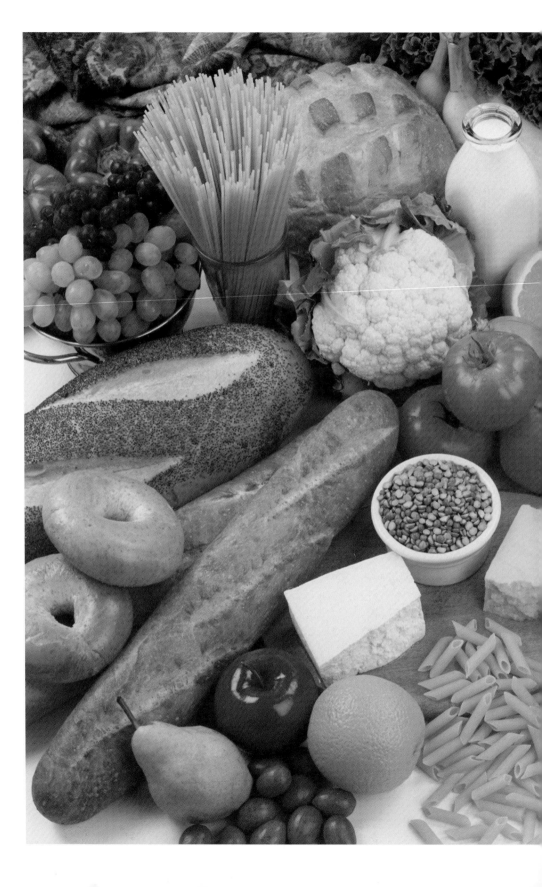

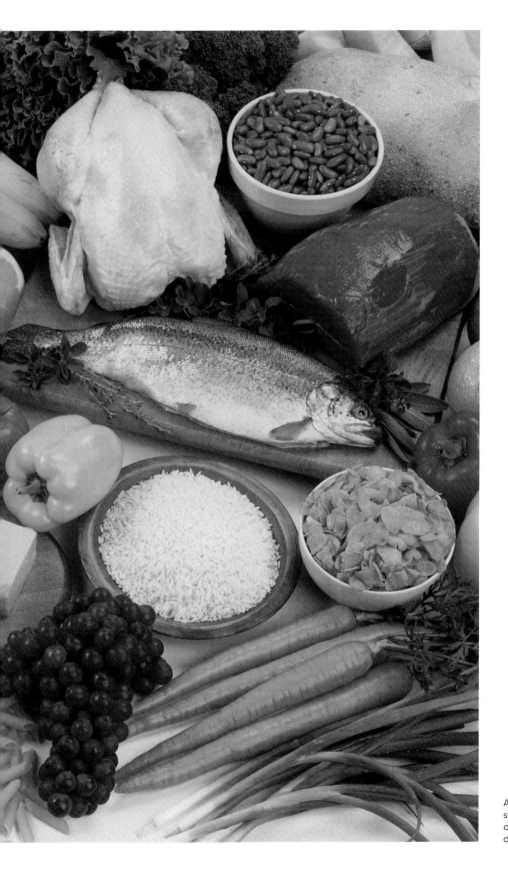

A balanced diet should take care of all your dietary needs

NUTRITION

EATING TO EXERCISE

Eating should be a relatively straightforward procedure. But for something so simple, we have managed to complicate the issue to such an extent that very few people now feel confident in selecting the right foods to fuel their everyday lives, let alone a lifestyle that includes demanding physical exercise.

Much of the confusion stems from the overwhelming array of nutritional extras like supplements, drinks, pills and potions designed to speed up the route to wellbeing. Many of them are specifically targeted at those who take part in regular exercise and manufacturers bombard us with claims that their latest offering is the product of rocket science, a fuel or supplement that will launch you into orbit.

If you don't consume it, they say, you are forever destined to be unfit and overweight; if you consume enough of it you will suddenly find you are blessed with the endurance capacities of Forrest Gump and the physique.

In fact, eating the right sort of diet to complement your lifestyle is far less complicated than some supplement manufacturers would have us believe.

What it boils down to is consuming enough of the right sorts of foods in the right amounts to provide enough energy to fuel whatever amount of exercise you choose to do. The trick is not to lose your way in the dietary maze. Here is a guide to taking the most direct route to a healthy diet:

Constructing your personal dietary plan

One thing that most experts agree on is that there is no one wonder diet that can be prescribed for everyone. The main reason for this is that our lifestyles, work patterns, activity levels, food preferences and digestive systems are unique to each of us and consequently there is never going to be one eating plan that suits all. The key to finding a diet that works for you ultimately boils down to analysing the structure of your own life. So get down to the nitty gritty:

LOOK AT YOUR SCHEDULE

Firstly, take a long hard look at your average daily patterns. What time do you get up? And go to bed? Is your work physical or are you stuck behind a desk all day? Do you regularly work through your lunch break and grab a snack or are you obliged to attend business lunches? And, importantly, at what time of day do you usually work out? Then write down the key timings of your daily schedule. Plan when is the best time for you to eat breakfast, lunch, evening meal and snacks. Determine when you are going to visit the gym or head out for a run and back-track to find the time two-to-three hours beforehand when you should eat a high carbohydrate snack. In much the same way as you plan your working week, get into the habit of mentally planning ahead as far as your diet is concerned.

WHAT DO YOU LIKE TO EAT?

For a healthy diet to be effective, it must be one that you can stick to and, therefore should consist of foods that you like eating. One common mistake is to stock up on foods that you think you should be eating only to discover that when it comes to the crunch and you are feeling ravenously hungry, you don't fancy munching on mung-bean and rocket salad, so order a high fat pepperoni pizza instead. Instead, stock your freezer and cupboards with quick to prepare foods that are wholesome and will satisfy your appetite as well as your tastebuds. Bagels, rice, noodles, crackers and pasta are good choices for store-cupboard carbohydrates; frozen vegetables and juices are a handy standby as are ready made sauces and low fat ready meals.

Change your bad habits

The simplest changes to your daily diet are often the most effective. Again, the best place to start is with a notepad in which you jot down your daily food and drink consumption for at least 24 hours – and no cheating. Every crumb of fruitcake, every broken biscuit and every gallon of cola should be recorded.

The results may surprise you. However, only when you can see plainly and clearly what you are doing wrong can you set about making it right. Perhaps you limp through the day on a very low fluid intake or snack on more high fat chocolate bars or crisps than you realised. With that in mind, make your own list of dietary resolutions to drink more fluid or eat more wholesome snacks like fruit.

How much and what type of carbohydrate do you need?

According to current Department of Health recommendations, the average person should aim to get 50 per cent of their calories from carbohydrate foods. For people who do a lot of exercise or have very active jobs, however, most sports nutritionists advise consuming between three and five grams of carbohydrate food for every pound of their body weight which equates to 60 to 70 per cent of your total calorie intake.

There are three main types of carbohydrate – sugars (simple carbohydrate), starches (complex) and fibre (complex) – all of which need to be consumed for a balanced diet. Ideally you should select foods that provide all three types of carbohydrate and not rely solely on one source. Complex carbohydrates are those found in starchy foods like pasta, bread and potatoes and are broken down by the body more slowly than sugars which are rapidly digested and absorbed.

Some sugars, like fructose (fruit sugar) and lactose (milk sugar) must first be converted into glucose before they can be used for energy which means they cannot be used quite as quickly for fuel. But, in general, simple carbohydrates are used to satisfy the body's more immediate energy requirements while complex carbohydrates are first converted into glycogen and then stored as an energy reserve.

Muscles can normally store enough glycogen to fuel from 90 minutes to two hours of physical activity but a high carbohydrate diet composed of both sugars and starches can increase the body's reserves and result in an improved capacity for endurance exercise. Typically, the average person who works out would need to consume the equivalent of the following daily food combinations to obtain adequate carbohydrate:

Example one: one bowl of cereal, 6 slices of wholemeal bread, 200 grams of boiled potatoes or a chickpea and bean salad, one slice of plain fruit cake, 1 apple, 1 banana, 1 pear and a slice of melon.

Example two: four thick slices of bread, 1 large jacket potato, 1 large portion of pasta or rice, 1 scone or 2 digestive biscuits, 1 banana, I orange and a small bunch of grapes.

THE QUICK FIX MIRACLE-MAKERS

Since what we eat is inextricably linked with the way we look and that, in turn, is closely related to varying levels of insecurity, it should come as no surprise to hear that the diet world is full of sharks waiting to pounce at times when you are feeling most vulnerable about your appearance.

There are plenty that claim ta quick fix miracle, even if they are scientifically unproven and possibly bad for you. So no wonder people everywhere are turning to:

The Cabbage Soup Diet
Enthusiasts claim you can lose up to 17lbs in one week which is hardly

surprising when your staple food is a watery green soup and your only other source of calories comes from vegetables (but no potatoes) and fruit (but no bananas). Still, it is one of the most popular diets of all time, even though for anyone remotely active it is a fast route to energy depletion.

Carbo-Unloading diet

The latest offering from the gym-obsessed Americans is a diet which claims to help you burn fat faster by exercising on an empty stomach and then fasting for a few hours afterwards. Basically you deny yourself any form of carbohydrate for at least three hours before a run and then hold out for as long as possible before eating anything when you finish. Professor Ian Macdonald, head of the School of Biomedical Sciences at Nottingham University, says that exercising with low glycogen stores is dangerous. "In the long term it will result in loss of muscle rather than body fat," he warns.

The Food Combining diet

Every few years a new version of the Hay Diet, devised at the beginning of century, surfaces and we are once again warned not to eat carbohydrates and protein at the same time and that we should eat the 'right' foods to restore the body's natural balance between acids and alkalis.

"There is no scientific evidence to support this theory whatsoever," says Professor Tom Sanders of the nutrition department at Kings College, London. "The rules are inherently contradictory and the whole idea of food combining is nutritional nonsense."

WHAT ABOUT SUPPLEMENTS?

Mention vitamins and minerals and supplements automatically spring to most people's minds. Latest figures show that 40 per cent of the population now regularly takes a nutritional supplement at a cost of £1million a day, with year on year sales rising from £180million in 1994 to an anticipated £500million by the end of next year. However, to date, neither the Department of Health (DoH) nor conventional nutritionists advocate routinely taking extra nutrients in the form of tablets and capsules as part of a healthy diet.

According to Gail Goldberg, a nutrition scientist at the British Nutrition Foundation, there are certain social groups who are considered to be at a higher risk of nutrient deficiency, including pregnant and breast-feeding women, faddy dieters, smokers and the elderly.

"These people may need some form of supplementation to their diets, but the rest of us should be able to get enough vitamins and minerals from the food we eat," she says.

"At present there is no conclusive evidence to support a general, healthy population taking nutritional supplements although that advice may change if new research emerges."

It is useful to check food labels to make sure that you are getting a sufficiently high nutrient intake. Most manufacturers now list vitamin and mineral content. You will usually find figures listed as a percentage of the Recommended Daily Amounts/Allowances (RDA) – an indication of the average necessary intake of a particular nutrient that people should aim to get from their food.

Although these are figures for the average adult and do not take into account activity levels or individual requirements they can be used as a rough guide. A Reference Nutrient Intake (RNI) is a figure which, according to the Department of Health, is set according to age and sex and one which should meet the nutritional needs of the majority of the UK population. Again, the figures should be used as a rough guide.

However, there are some vitamin and mineral supplements that experts agree are beneficial for certain groups:

Multivitamin

If in doubt, choose a good quality multivitamin from a health food store, not a supermarket where the quality is variable, and look for a product that provides the recommended daily amount (RDA) of a number of nutrients. Generally the more you spend on a multivitamin, the better quality you get.

Calcium

The National Osteoporosis Society recommends an intake of 800mg a day (1000mg for teenagers). If you don't eat dairy foods, the supplement might be worthwhile.

Vitamin D

Also important in the prevention of brittle bones. It is produced when your skin is exposed to sunlight, so if you spend all your time indoors you may need to get ten micrograms of vitamin D from food and a supplement could help.

Vitamin B12

Vegetarians may need a supplement of B12 (around 1.5 micrograms a day) since the best source is meat and animal products.

Folic Acid

The Department of Health recommends that all women planning a pregnancy take a daily supplement of 400 micrograms of folic acid (and continue to do so for the first 12 weeks of pregnancy) to lower the risk of neural tube defects in their unborn child. High levels of folic acid have recently been linked to the lowering of homocysteine levels in the blood, a substance that is thought to increase the risk of heart disease.

A GUIDE TO FITNESS SUPPLEMENTS

For your every physical weakness, there is a now a pill or potion in a bottle that manufacturers claim will rectify it. These supplements are usually made from natural substances and do not feature on UK Sport's list of banned substances. But the million dollar question is, do they work?

Creatine

Creatine is a naturally-occurring compound found in meat and fish and stored in the body's muscles. It is used to generate energy and power muscles in intense bursts of physical activity lasting from one to ten seconds. Almost 150 clinical studies have proven that supplements of Creatine can help to boost performance in sports which involve some fast sprinting.

There is also evidence that it helps prevent the build-up of lactic acid during exercise. However, UK Sport's Ethics and Anti-Doping department say the evidence for the safe use of creatine is insubstantial. There are concerns about possible damage to the liver and kidneys with large doses of Creatine.

Chromium

This trace mineral is found naturally in nuts, cheese and wholegrains. One of its main roles is to help insulin transport blood sugar into muscle cells. In supplement form it is usually sold as chromium picolinate (picolinate is a metal that helps the body absorb chromium) with claims that it will enhance fat-burning . Early studies carried out ten years ago suggested this might be the case.

However, latest research suggests chromium supplements offer very few benefits unless you are deficient in the mineral anyway. One US study in 1996 showed that 24-year-old men who followed a weight training schedule for 12 weeks improved their strength by 23 per cent when they took a daily supplement of chromium, but that was ten per cent LESS than subjects who took nothing at all.

Conjugated Linoleic Acid (CLA)

CLA is naturally present in animal foods like beef and dairy products.

Studies on animals found that it helped to increase lean body mass. It has been the subject of a few clinical trials on humans which suggest it assists the body in using its energy stores more effectively and helps regulate the storage of body fat.

One double blind study showed that subjects who took a daily CLA supplement for three months achieved an average 15 to 20 per cent reduction in body fat percentages compared with those who took a placebo. But most experts are wary that studies have been carried out only on animals using high doses of CLA and its benefits for humans have yet to be confirmed. Unless water consumption is increased when you take it, CLA may also result in dehydration.

L-Carnitine

This is an amino acid that is made naturally in the liver and is involved in transporting fat across cells into the muscle where it is used for energy. The theory is that, the more carnitine you consume, the more fat you will break down during exercise. Proponents claim that, because it may help fat to be used more efficiently as a fuel, it will improve endurance levels.

Some small studies have suggested it can help reduce muscle soreness after a workout. But the majority of studies show it to have no benefit on either fat transportation or helping to get rid of body fat. A study of marathon runners in 1996 showed that those who took supplements of L-Carnitine before and after a race did not improve their performance, recovery time or fat-burning levels.

Pyruvate

This is a compound that occurs naturally in the body and is used to help convert blood sugar into glycogen, the main fuel for aerobic exercise. Some studies, including one at the University of Pittsburgh in 1992, have shown that taking high doses of pyruvate in supplement form may help reduce body fat and endurance without the need to exercise. It has also been suggested that it may enable you to work out more often. But to date, studies have been carried out on obese women taking huge doses of pyruvate (up to 100 grams a day) who are also following a calorie restrictive diet.

Experts are concerned about the effect such high intakes can have on the delicate balance of minerals and body salts. In 1997, researchers at the University of Memphis showed that daily supplementation with pyruvate by a group of overweight women resulted in them losing only one pound a month more than counterparts who didn't take it.

SPORTS DRINKS
Are they Worth the Money?

Top athletes and footballers are rarely spotted without a bottle containing the latest sports drink. According to the manufacturers, they not only boost energy but may also improve performance and endurance levels when you exercise.

There are basically two kinds of sports drink, both containing small particles of easily absorbed carbohydrate. The isotonic drinks have the same osmolality (or concentration of dissolved particles) as the body's own fluids, are therefore easily absorbed and are designed to be taken both during, before and after exercise. Hypotonic drinks, on the other hand, have fewer particles than the body's own fluids and are absorbed faster than plain water.

Research has proven that sports drinks can be beneficial to performance – but only in activities lasting longer than 90 minutes. Anything less than that and the main aim is simply to replace fluid lost through sweat to avoid dehydration and plain old water will do the job perfectly well. In endurance events like the marathon, drinks containing between four and eight per cent of carbohydrate particles can improve stamina.

Many also contain small amounts of sodium which enhances fluid absorption. In fact, studies on marathon runners who take commercially prepared sports drinks, as opposed to water, have shown that they have a higher total fluid consumption.

WHERE TO GO FOR HELP

If you feel uneasy about your diet and want help devising an eating plan that will work just for you then it is important to consult an expert. Beware that anyone can set themselves up as a nutritionist although qualifications can vary from a certificate awarded for a one-day course to a postgraduate university degree. So who should you choose?

The dietitian

"A State Registered Dietitian (SRD) has been clinically trained and has completed either a four year degree in dietetics or a science degree (perhaps nutrition) followed by a two year postgraduate qualification," says Haydn Hughes of the British Dietetic Association (BDA). Only SRDs are employed within the NHS and they follow the official medical guidelines issued by the Department of Health.

You can be referred to the SRD at your local hospital by your GP, but usually only if she or he has diagnosed a problem. Alternatively, you can see an SRD privately for advice. The BDA keeps a register of qualified dietitians in the UK. Send an SAE to BDA, Fifth Floor, Elizabeth House, 22 Suffolk Street, Queensway, Birmingham, B1 1LS (0121 616 4900).

The Nutritionist

As it stands the law does not prohibit anyone from calling themselves a nutritionist, so always check out qualifications beforehand. Look for a degree in nutrition and some post-graduate experience. Typically a nutritionist won't advocate the use of supplements unless you have a vitamin or mineral deficiency and will work to help you get the most out of the food you eat. The British Nutrition Foundation (0207 404

6504) has experts on hand to answer telephone queries about diet or for more general information, consult their website at www.nutrition.org.uk

The Sports Nutritionist

For more specific advice about nutrition for sport, it is worth consulting a sports nutrition expert. The Sports Nutrition Foundation at the National Sports Medicine Institute in London runs an accredited sports nutrition course for anyone who is already an SRD. For details contact the institute on 0207 251 0583

The Personal Trainer

Although the average gym instructor or personal trainer is versed in the benefits of physical training and a healthy lifestyle, in most cases they are not qualified to give nutritional advice. If they claim to have a qualification, it is worth investigating which one. Many gyms and health clubs run in-house courses.

The Nutrition Therapist

A nutrition therapist aims to prevent and treat problems using a range of dietary techniques including the use of supplements, elimination diets and intolerance testing. Once more, the qualifications vary considerably and none are recognised by the BDA or the BNF. Still, if this approach is for you, contact the Society for the Promotion of Nutritional Therapy, PO Box 47, Heathfield, East Sussex, TN21 8ZX for more information.

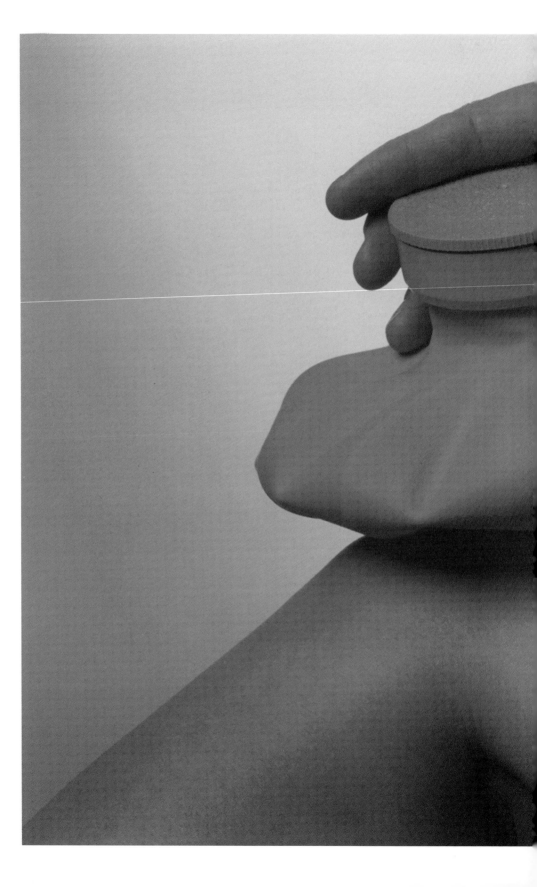

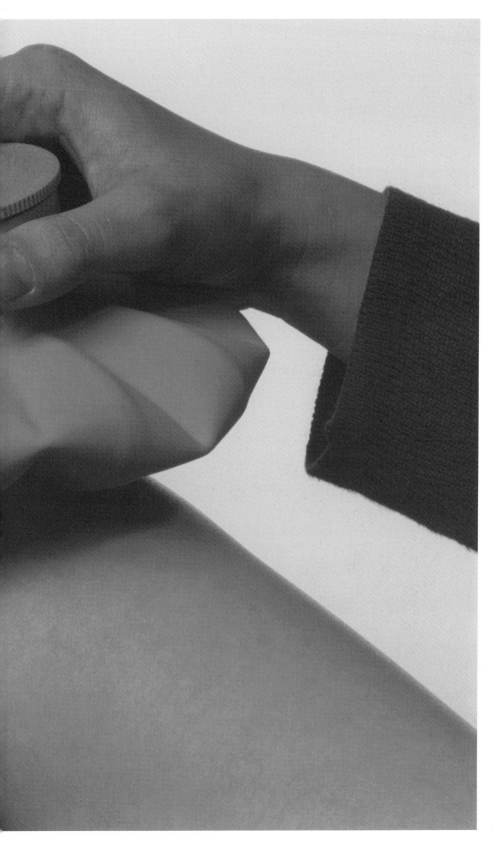

INJURIES & PROBLEMS

Remember 'RICE'

INJURIES & PROBLEMS

INJURIES

Every year in the UK, the total number of sports injuries exceeds 20 million and that is despite increasing knowledge about how best to warm-up and cool down before and after exercise. Getting injured can be a blow to your fitness programme, but knowing how to treat and care for an injury could have you back up and running much sooner.

According to physiotherapists, there are basically four types of injury and treatments will vary according to their severity. Muscle soreness usually lasts 24 to 48 hours and is caused by tiny tears to the muscle fibres resulting in soreness around the affected muscle. Slightly more severe are muscle strains the result of more tears to fibres and causing pain on movement that can restrict range of motion.

A bad muscle strain can take months to heal properly while a minor strain can be repaired in weeks. Acute injuries cause pain that will prevent you from exercising and may require the attention of a chartered physiotherapist while the most enduring chronic injuries can persist for months, even years and affect overall performance, technique or style in sport.

What you do immediately after any injury, however minor, will have a huge influence on how long it will last. Injury to a part of the body will cause inflammation and soreness and the easiest and most effective way to reduce this is to apply ice to the affected area as soon as you can. All physiotherapists drum in the importance of the acronym R.I.C.E.: rest, ice, compression and elevation to speed up recovery.

Clare Doyle, chartered sports physiotherapist at the London Clinic, suggests a simple plan of action to self-treat a minor injury: Start by applying an ice pack to the affected area. Always wrap ice or a packet of frozen vegetables, like peas, in a tea towel and apply intermittently for a few minutes at a time to avoid burning your skin. Do this for ten to 15 minutes. Next, if necessary, apply compression with a bandage that is tight, but does not restrict circulation.

This helps to reduce swelling and internal bleeding. Finally, try to keep the injured part of your body elevated which allows the fluid causing the swelling to drain away. Rest for at least 48 hours or until you can comfortably use the joint again.

Who to Contact: To find a chartered sports physiotherapist in your area, call PhysioFirst on 01327 354441. For information on avoiding sports injuries visit the Chartered Society of Physiotherapy website at www.csp.org.uk; the National Sports Medicine Institute can be contacted on 0207 251 0583.

MOTIVATIONAL SLUMPS

A few years ago a national campaign to get us off our sofas and up exercising used the slogan "the hardest thing about getting fit is getting started." What it failed to mention was that staying fit involves a fair bit of effort too. The very fitness programme that seemed such a good idea when you first jogged a lap of the park, kick boxed your way through a class or paddled a few lengths of the local pool can lose its appeal when the weather gets colder, work gets more stressful or when you don't seem to be losing weight as quickly as you thought you would.

Sad to say, most newly-pledged vows of fitness are broken within the first year, while 60 per cent of gym members throw in the towel less than six months after forking out their registration fee. But what is it that sets the exercise recidivists aside from the committed enthusiast who manages to get fit and stay fit? The answer is motivation. If you can train your mind at the same time as getting your body into shape, nothing will stand in your way:

Make friends with your body: Trying to get fit will be a constant struggle if you think of your body as an enemy that needs to be punished. Take a good look at yourself in the mirror and learn to deal with your body as it is now; check out your good points and try to accept any imperfections. People who get depressed about the way they look are more likely to get caught in a vicious cycle of skipping workouts and then comforting themselves with food.

Get fit for yourself: Before you make a commitment to get fit, make sure you are doing it for the right reasons. Do it because you want to feel good about yourself, not because someone has criticised you for being unfit. Similarly, if you decide to get fit simply to lose weight, you will probably find that the inspiration dwindles once you have reached your target weight. An external motive like fitting into a skimpy outfit means you are less likely to keep up the good work – so shape up for yourself, nothing else.

You don't have to do it: Always remember that whatever way you decide to keep fit, it is supposed to be fun. Some people develop a misguided sense of duty and feel obliged to carry on exactly as they started. But if you don't enjoy what you are doing – don't do it! Try something different or if you usually work out alone, try exercising with a group. A change can be a refreshing way to rekindle your enthusiasm.

Just one step... If cold weather is making you reluctant to leave your living room or you simply don't feel like exercising, try telling yourself that you will just do ten minutes of running instead of 20 or 15 minutes of an aerobics class instead of the whole thing. By the time you have done the small amount you will probably have found the incentive to carry on.

Stay on track: Nobody's pretending that staying fit is easy all the time. There will be days when you will feel too tired to do anything or times when commitments to your family, partner or job disrupt your exercise programme. But that is the nature of the beast. The key is not to dwell on missed workouts and to put them behind as soon as you can. You don't become unfit overnight. Longer term problems may require you to reassess your goals and develop a revised, less-demanding schedule. Don't worry if this happens to you. You are not a failure just because you have to adjust your expectations.

Plan ahead: One of the best ways to keep motivated is to set regular goals for yourself. Plan ahead and jot down what you want to achieve from your workouts. Writing something in a diary or note pad means that, subconsciously, you have already made a commitment to yourself.

Maybe you want to run a regular route in a certain time, or cycle for ten minutes longer than usual. One of the main goals of exercise is to finish feeling you have achieved something and there is always something to aim for. Don't go out and exercise aimlessly.

Accentuate the positive: Just as exercising regularly week after week will eventually make you physically more powerful, so repeatedly focussing on your strengths and achievements will leave you psychologically stronger. Years of telling yourself that you can't get fit or lose weight could mean that you have made a habit of thinking negatively, but you can change that by proving yourself wrong. As you get fitter, focus on your success – landmarks of any size – and watch your self confidence grow.

ADDICTED TO EXERCISE

Exercise addiction is commonly referred to as the newest self-inflicted disorder of our time by psychologists. While most of us still don't work out often enough to satisfy health experts, an increasing number of men and women can't stop exercising. Typically they set themselves punishing daily schedules and restrict the number of calories they consume in their diet to a minimum.

Researchers at the University of Birmingham's School of Sport and Exercise Science are currently studying the link between exercise addiction and eating disorders. Diane Bamber, one of the researchers, says that what starts as as healthy commitment to exercise can become an unhealthy obsession. More and more people, she says, are losing control of their fitness goals and, consequently, are developing eating disorders such as anorexia and bulimia nervosa.

According to the University of Birmingham researchers, there are signs that you are developing an unhealthy obsession with exercise. Answer yes to any of these questions and you may need to revaluate your reasons for working out or even to seek professional help:

1. Do you stick to an inflexible exercise programme?
2. Do you plan your day around your workout?
3. Do you suffer withdrawal symptoms when you are forced to miss a workout?
4. Does exercise interfere with your work or social life?
5. Does exercise cause problems with your personal relationships?

Who to Contact: Treatment is not straightforward and the biggest stumbling block with an eating disorder or exercise addiction is usually denial by the person that it exists at all. However, once someone has accepted they are over-dependent on exercise, the first step is to seek help.

Talk to family and friends if you can, but otherwise contact a professional, like your GP. The Eating Disorders Association's help line is on 01603 621414; Runner's World magazine runs a self-help network and can put you in touch with an exercise psychologist or dietitian. Send an SAE to the Buddy Scheme, Runner's World, 7-10 Chandos Street, London, W1M OAD.

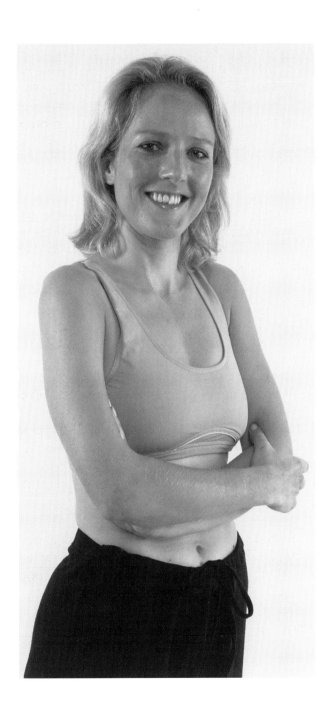

OTHER USEFUL NUMBERS

British Dance Council
Terpsichore House,
240 Merton Road,
London, SW19 1EQ
(0208 5450085)

British Slimnastics Association
Chiltern Vale,
16 Foxtell Way,
Chalfont St Peter,
Bucks, SL9 OPN
(01494
873576)

British Wheel of Yoga
1 Hamilton Place,
Boston road,
Sleaford,
Lincs, NG34 7ES
(01529 306851)

Exercise England
Solecast House,
13-27 Brunswick Place,
London N1 6DX
(0870 750 6506)

Keep Fit Association
Francis House,
Francis Street,
London, SW1P 1DE
(0207 233 8898)
email: user@thekfa.doctornet.co.uk

English Folk Dance and Song Society
Cecil Sharp House,
2 Regents Park Road,
London, NW1 7AY
(0207 485 2206)
www.efdss.org.co

The British Hang-gliding and Paragliding Association
The Old Schoolroom,
Loughborough Road,
Leicestershire, LE4 5PJ
(0116 261 1322)

British Sub-Aqua Club
Telfords Quay,
Ellesmere Port,
South Wirral,
Cheshire, L65 4FY
(0151 3507 6200)

British Water Ski Federation
390 City Road,
London, EC1V 2QA
(0207 833 2855 ext 22)
email: info@bwsf.co.uk